SELF-HELP FOR

Hyperventilation Syndrome

*Recognizing and Correcting
Your Breathing-Pattern Disorder*

Third Revised Edition

DINAH BRADLEY

D1115455

> Hunter House Inc., Publishers
> PO Box 2914
> Alameda CA 94501-0914

Library of Congress Cataloging-in-Publication Data
Bradley, Dinah.
    Self-help for hyperventilation syndrome : recognizing and correcting your breathing-pattern disorder / Dinah Bradley.— 3rd rev. ed.
        p. cm.
    Includes bibliographical references and index.
    ISBN 0-89793-348-6 (pa) — ISBN 0-89793-349-4 (cl)
        1. Hyperventilation. 2. Hyperventilation—Psychosomatic aspects.
3. Stress management. I. Title.
RC776.H9 B733 2001
616.2'08—dc21   2001026468

Project Credits

Cover Design: Brian Dittmar
Illustrations: Sally Hollis-McLeod
Proofreader: John David Marion
Acquisitions Editor: Jeanne Brondino
Associate Editor:
  Alexandra Mummery
Editorial and Production Assistant:
  Emily Tryer
Administrator: Theresa Nelson
Computer Support:
  Peter Eichelberger
Publisher: Kiran S. Rana

Book Design and Production:
  Jinni Fontana
Copy Editor: Kelley Blewster
Indexer: Kathy Talley-Jones
Publicity Manager: Sara Long
Acquisitions and Publicity Assistant:
  Lori Covington
Sales and Marketing Assistant:
  Earlita K. Chenault
Customer Service Manager:
  Christina Sverdrup
Order Fulfillment: Joel Irons

Printed and Bound by Bang Printing, Brainerd, Minnesota
Manufactured in the United States of America

9 8 7 6 5 4 3 2 1   3rd Revised Edition   01 02 03 04 05

CONTENTS

FOREWORD

Modern technology has afforded mankind a host of advantages. It has become possible to travel the world rapidly, communicate almost instantaneously over long distances via the Internet, microwave a meal in seconds, commute to work in a climate-controlled car listening to digitally reproduced classical music. Advances in medicine and public health have controlled many diseases and prolonged the average human life span to record levels. Yet in spite of these advances, and in part because of them, the pace of human life has accelerated, resulting in ever-increasing levels of psychological stress.

The effects of this stress manifest in a variety of ways. The body adapts to high levels of stress with different responses. Some are beneficial (e.g., a greater alertness or arousal state), but many are detrimental. Examples of maladaptive responses to stress include posttraumatic stress disorder, certain types of headache, and perhaps even peptic ulcers and coronary artery disease. Mental disorders such as agoraphobia, panic disorder, and many varieties of neurosis are either caused by, or at least exacerbated by, high levels of stress. As daily functioning is progressively impaired by anxiety, depression commonly results. Hyperventilation syndrome in both its acute and chronic forms is one of the maladaptive responses to stress that has become a silent epidemic. It is epidemic because so many people are affected, and it is silent because the syndrome is so seldom recognized by the clinicians to whom sufferers turn.

Acute hyperventilation consists of overbreathing to the point where body chemistry is disrupted, and the typical symptoms consist of tingling in the hands and around the mouth, confusion and panic because of diminished blood flow to the brain, a sensation of inability to take a deep breath, palpitations, tremor, sweating ... in short, a sensation that death by asphyxiation is imminent. While the acute hyperventilation syndrome is usually correctly diagnosed, it is often dismissed by clinicians as something less than a real disease like pulmonary embolism or myocardial infarction. The patient is reassured that nothing serious is wrong and is prescribed sedatives or left to his or her own devices to prevent recurrences. Unfortunately, the patient experiences real agony with this condition and recurrences are common.

Chronic hyperventilation syndrome (HVS) is a much more common and subtler condition. There is no overt rapid breathing and no classic constellation of symptoms that lead to rapid diagnosis. It may present with substernal chest pain reminiscent of angina, feelings of dizziness or faintness, difficulty breathing, and a host of neurologic symptoms. It is estimated that approximately 10 percent of general Internal Medicine and Family Practice patients are suffering from chronic hyperventilation syndrome. Admission to hospital for investigation of possible cardiac or neurologic disorders is extremely common and many patients with chronic HVS carry an assortment of incorrect diagnoses with bottles of corresponding ineffective medications. Apart from the expense of these investigations, unnecessary medications, and time lost from work, there is a small but real risk associated with certain medical investigations such as angiography and from the side effects of medications.

The medical community has failed patients with HVS. It has failed to recognize the very real agony that these patients suffer and the negative impact it has on their lives. It has failed to establish clear diagnostic criteria for HVS. Most importantly, it has failed to recognize that there are simple, effective treatments for HVS. The treatments described in this text are simple. Once learned, they can be practiced almost anywhere a patient might find his or herself. However, as HVS is a learned, maladaptive response to stress, it takes a commitment to relearn proper breathing techniques and patience on the part of the patient and the therapist to completely reverse the condition.

Dinah Bradley has written a clear, easily understood explanation of the causes and manifestations of HVS. She has outlined a rehabilitative program that will be instructive for therapists but that can also easily be practiced by patients on their own. If you recognize yourself in these pages, start practicing these simple breathing techniques. Over a relatively short time you will find your attacks becoming less frequent and less severe until hyperventilation becomes a memory rather than an incapacitating burden.

— Edward Newton, M.D., FACEP

PREFACE

My sister lent me an earlier edition of this book several years ago. I put it in my "to read later" pile, and thought nothing more of it. A year later—2 weeks before my 21st birthday— I landed in the hospital as the result of a nasty combination of a chest infection, anemia, the inevitable "change of season," and my long-term asthma.

When I was first diagnosed with asthma and given the sticky, sugary Ventolin syrup, I was told I would grow out of it in my teens. My doctor also said, "Breathe through your nose." I tried. It was uncomfortable. I gave up. That was the only practical advice that anyone ever gave me, other than to take my medicine regularly.

Until that major attack, I had tried to ignore my asthma, although, looking back, there was no way I could. I was bound to it. I would feel powerless and panicky if I found myself somewhere without my inhaler, and I had no reliable method to calm myself down. Graduating to steroid "preventers" made it worse because now I had two inhalers to lug everywhere. And to use an inhaler in public felt like I was admitting to those around me that I was unfit and unhealthy—even though I have always been a regular exerciser.

Although the hospital episode was a miserable and painful one, it was also the turning point in my attitude to my asthma. Interestingly, it wasn't being in the hospital that panicked me. I was warm and well looked after, apart from the chain-smoking doctor who, without asking, trundled in with 10 medical students, tried to convince me it was psychosomatic, and let me know that asthma gets worse for women in their early 20s.

The panic came when it was time to leave. Our house was being renovated, there was sawdust everywhere, and that scared me. It was a windy day outside and that scared me.

The idea of dancing at my 21st birthday party scared me. The thought of setting foot inside a smoky bar terrified me, let alone getting to the end of a sentence in my broadcasting job. In short, in the hospital, the medical staff and oxygen masks were in control of my lungs. Outside, it was just me.

After 21 years of letting other people (not) tell me what to do, and being a slave to my inhaler, I had developed a strong sense that there must be another way for me to gain power over my asthma. And since no one was offering, I had to ask around. At the asthma clinic where I'd been referred I asked if there was some sort of breathing specialist. That's when I met Dinah Bradley.

As we worked on my breathing technique, I remembered many things from the past: the doctor who told me to breathe through my nose; acting classes where we had to "breathe into our stomachs"; the reason I got so tired during clothes-shopping expeditions ("Hold your tummies in, girls!"). They were all things that made perfect sense, but I had to discover them for myself because my experiences with the medical world were so, well, medicine-focused.

I cured my penchant for yawning, and I learned how to breathe my way out of minor asthmatic irritations. I'm no longer scared to go anywhere or do anything, and if I am caught somewhere without my inhaler, I can calm myself with my breathing, rather than let my breathing panic me (or I could just ask the one in three New Zealand families who use one to borrow an inhaler).

I consider other improvements in my life—sleeping well, regular exercise, no more depression, increased self-confidence, and a generally happy disposition—to be a direct result of better breathing. It's the most fundamental of our human functions, and it's not until you can't take it for granted that you truly appreciate it. Best thing is, it's free.

Strangely, I only ever get panic attacks now when I see Dinah. I nervously check my breathing, make sure my posture is relaxed, and watch the imaginary bag of rice rise and fall. Why do I get nervous? Because she's one of the two women who changed my life. I'm the other one.

It is so important to be your own health expert. I strongly urge you to take control of your own health, ask as many questions as you have to, explore every option available to you. And if someone gives you this book—read it!

— Gemma Gracewood
Editorial Director, Radio 95 FM
Auckland, New Zealand

ACKNOWLEDGMENTS

Heartfelt appreciation to Hunter House for publishing a North American edition of this book, with very special thanks to the editorial team for its guidance and support.

I would like to acknowledge the original and groundbreaking work of British physician Claude Lum, MA, MB, FRCP, FRACP, in reexamining this "ubiquitous disorder" and inspiring continued clinical research into breathing and respiratory dysfunction as well as British physiotherapists Diana Innocenti and Rosemary Cluff for their seminal work in the treatment of chronic hyperventilators.

I wish to express my gratitude and thanks to Edward Newton, M.D., Vice Chairman, Associate Professor of Emergency Medicine, Los Angeles County/University of Southern California Medical Center, for generously agreeing to write the North American foreword.

To my physiotherapy colleagues, especially my practice partner at B r e a t h i n g Works, Tania Clifton-Smith—warmest thanks for your support and help.

Many thanks to the physicians who now include breathing-pattern disorders in their diagnostic repertoire. Particular thanks to John Henley, MB, ChB, FRACP, for professional kindness and support.

Special thanks to Sally Hollis-McLeod for her splendid drawings.

To Victoria University Press, my appreciation for permission to use an extract from *The Miserables*, by Damien Wilkins.

Finally, a salute to the many hundreds of patients ranging in age from 5 to 88 years, from all races, genders, and creeds, who have helped me experiment, research, and shape the BETTER Breathing Plan.

— *Dinah Bradley, Dip. Phys., NZRP, MNZSP*

IMPORTANT NOTE

The material in this book is intended to provide a review of resources and information related to hyperventilation syndrome/breathing-pattern disorders. Every effort has been made to provide accurate and dependable information. However, professionals in the field may have differing opinions and change is always taking place. Any of the treatments described herein should be undertaken only under the guidance of a licensed health-care practitioner. The author, editors, and publishers cannot be held responsible for any error, omission, professional disagreement, outdated material, or adverse outcomes that derive from use of any of these treatments or information resources in this book, either in a program of self-care or under the care of a licensed practitioner.

INTRODUCTION

In the 10 years since I wrote the first edition of this book, many, many people have written to tell me, or have told me in person, how much they appreciate its message.

It seemed to hit the right buttons for the huge group of people who suffered from this mysterious and then little-known stress disorder.

This third, expanded edition is a result of lobbying from patients wanting more comments and stories from other patients. Still others requested a workbook section to help them keep track of their progress; this is included at the back of the book.

Hyperventilation syndrome—HVS—has been used as a descriptive title since the mid-1930s, but it has been under intense scrutiny during the last decade. Some clinicians prefer the term *breathing-pattern disorders*. In this edition I use both terms.

Learning about normal breathing patterns and balanced body chemistry is one aspect of recovery. Getting the chest muscles, neck, and spine relaxed and working properly is another. Whether you can do this by yourself, or whether you need expert help, reading *Self-Help for Hyperventilation Syndrome* will help you sort out your priorities. Check with a physical therapist (known in New Zealand, Australia, and the United Kingdom as a physiotherapist, or respiratory physiotherapist). If you don't already work with a physical therapist who is familiar with this problem, ask your general practitioner to refer you to one.

We live in a stressed out world, and one thing stress is extremely good at is disturbing many of our vital body systems. Breathing is not exempt. All too often, after stressful events are over, many sufferers are left with habitually disordered breathing—HVS/BPDs—which are major sources of stress *all by themselves.*

Right in front of our nose floats the best antistress remedy imaginable—calm, energy-efficient breathing. Take the time to learn about this fascinating and complex process. It's the best investment you can make in reducing harmful stress levels, revitalizing your mind and body, and enjoying the gift of the breath of life to its fullest.

PART I

All About Hyperventilation Syndrome

CHAPTER 1

What Is Hyperventilation?

You have to breathe to live. But if you breathe too much, life becomes dominated by fear of symptoms, and fear of living life to its fullest.

— *Mike, 33*

The term *hyperventilation* means moving more air through the chest than the body can deal with. Most people have experienced hyperventilation—also called *overbreathing*—to some degree, usually in the form of an acute attack. It's a normal reaction to sudden danger or excitement, and the signs are easy to identify:

♦ Breathing and heart rate speed up

♦ Adrenaline pours into the bloodstream

♦ The nervous system is on "red alert"

♦ Muscles tense up

Sometimes people faint or collapse—or find superhuman reservoirs of strength. When the stressful event is over, the body returns to its normal relaxed state.

Less easy to spot is chronic hyperventilation, a breathing-pattern disorder in which overbreathing becomes a habit—usually in response to prolonged stress or tension. More widespread symptoms are felt, and at times these appear out of the blue. The symptoms may mimic serious disease or remind the sufferer of the perhaps frightening events surrounding a past acute attack. When this happens, more widespread symptoms mysteriously occur, such as the following:

THE CASCADE OF SYMPTOMS

```
ORIGINAL CAUSE
(psychological or physical stress)
        ▼
TENSION AND ANXIETY
        ▼
HYPERVENTILATION
        ▼
HYPERVENTILATION ATTACK
        ▼
ANTICIPATION ANXIETY
        ▼
POSSIBLE AVOIDANCE BEHAVIORS
```

- Breathlessness at rest for no apparent reason
- Frequent deep sighs or yawning
- Chest-wall pains
- Palpitations
- Light-headedness and feeling "spaced out"
- Tingling or numb lips or extremities
- Upset stomach or irritable bowel syndrome
- Achy muscles or joints, or tremors
- Tiredness, weakness, broken sleep, and nightmares
- Sexual problems
- Clammy hands and high anxiety or phobias

AUTONOMIC NERVOUS SYSTEM—
CONTROLLER OF INVOLUNTARY BODY FUNCTIONS

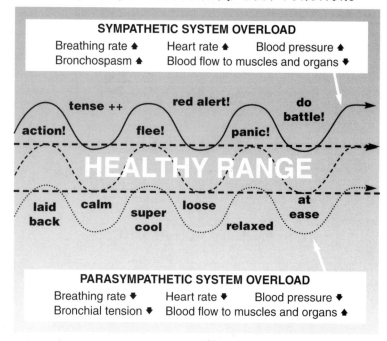

When overbreathing becomes chronic, the balance between the oxygen-rich air we breathe in and the carbon dioxide-rich air we breathe out is upset: carbon dioxide levels start to drop.

Far from being just a waste gas at the end of the respiratory cycle, carbon dioxide is a powerful governor of many of the body's systems—including blood flow to the brain. With chronic overbreathing the normal acid/alkaline balance (pH) of the tissues is altered. The body becomes more alkaline, and the nerve cells are the first to respond to this respiratory alkalosis. Dizziness and tingling or numbness are often the first signs.

The autonomic nervous system, which looks after the body's involuntary functions (for example, heart rate, blood pressure, and digestion), is affected, too. This system is di-

THE CAUSES OF CHRONIC HYPERVENTILATION

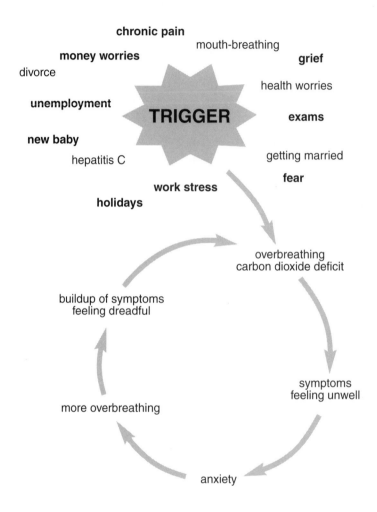

vided into two: the sympathetic, which governs action and "get up and go"; and the parasympathetic, which is responsible for rest, recuperation, and calmness. Low carbon dioxide levels stimulate the sympathetic nervous system more than the parasympathetic, putting the body on continuous red alert.

If carbon dioxide levels in the blood fall further with continued overbreathing, body cells begin to produce lactic acid in an effort to balance their pH. Muscles ache. Metabolism is less efficient. Exhaustion and chronic tiredness soon follow, with feelings of physical and mental depression—all typical signs of long-term chronic hyperventilation.

Not only nerve cells are affected. Muscle cells become more twitchy, and the smooth muscles of our blood vessels, airways, and gut tighten and constrict in response to lowered carbon dioxide. There is an increased release of histamines, which aggravates allergic responses. The heart starts pounding, and the hyperventilator may feel panic-stricken, with palpitations and feelings of "air hunger."

When carbon dioxide levels are too low, oxygen clings to its carriers—the red blood cells—and tissues, especially the brain, become starved of oxygen. The brain may have its oxygen supply cut by as much as 50 percent, making it difficult to concentrate, let alone feel like a part of this planet. The drop in oxygen supply to the brain stimulates the breathing-control center to increase breathing rates, and the chronic nature of the hyperventilation is reinforced.

Since the oxygen and carbon dioxide exchanges fuel every cell in our body, every system is ultimately going to be affected—leading to a distressing as well as puzzling range of symptoms.

Why Does Chronic Hyperventilation Happen?

Overbreathing is a normal reaction to stress or strain; it only becomes abnormal when stresses and strains reach levels that lead to chronic hyperventilation and outbreaks of symptoms. These stresses and strains may have started from:

- ◆ organic causes, for example, asthma, physical pain, pneumonia, anemia, chronic chest or heart disease;

♦ physiological causes, for example, fever, high progesterone levels, prolonged talking, high altitude, diabetes, liver or kidney disease;

♦ psychological and social causes, for example, fear, anxiety, depression, perfectionist personality, separation/divorce;

♦ unemployment or loneliness;

♦ drugs, for example, nicotine, caffeine, aspirin, amphetamines.

While these *original* causes may be dealt with, stabilized, or cured, in certain people the respiratory center in the brain is reset and the overbreathing becomes habitual. Even though the bad times are over, the increased breathing rate stays.

Worldwide, the last decade has been one of change and uncertainty. Our minds evolved in an ancestral environment that lacked the pressure, noise, and speed of the present electronic age. We're constantly bombarded with information and our brains often can't cope with it all. We need to consciously take time out to counter this megastimulation, but few of us do.

The increase in stress disorders and diseases is alarming. Computerization has pinned many workers in front of screens for extended periods of time, but the human body is not designed for prolonged sitting. We experience maximum stimulation from minimum effort, and breathing is affected.

Adapting to rapid change is especially difficult if the change is unwanted or out of our personal control. Stress levels soar, and with them adrenaline levels and heart rate, and nervous exhaustion follows—all fueled by overactive lungs.

Is Hyperventilation a Modern Disorder?

For centuries philosophers and scientists have understood the importance of good breathing. Hippocrates, the father of Western medicine, noted in the fifth century B.C., "The brain exercises the greatest power in mankind—but the air supplies sense to it."

Adherents of both Buddhism, which originated in India also in the fifth century B.C., and Taoism, from ancient China, combined breathing with relaxation and exercise to harmonize heart rate, breathing, digestion, and circulation. Yoga and t'ai chi are modern versions of these ancient wisdoms.

Despite well-observed accounts in Western literature of "breathless" heroines, or of heroes with their "breath taken away," little was understood about the link between over-breathing and ill health. The first detailed medical description of hyperventilation was not published until 1871, in a study of 300 American Civil War soldiers. A doctor noticed "disabling shortness of breath, irritable heart and oppression of breathing" and thought the cause of these problems lay in the heart.

Around the turn of the century, other medical researchers experimented with normal subjects, asking them to hyperventilate voluntarily; their results noted neurological effects (tingling and muscles spasms) as well.

The term *hyperventilation syndrome* (HVS) was coined in the 1930s. One British physician called it "one of the commonest chronic afflictions of sedentary town dwellers." Breathing into a paper bag (re-inhaling carbon dioxide-rich air) became a popular treatment for acute attacks of HVS.

No theater would be without a paper bag in the wings ready for stage-fright victims, frozen in respiratory alkalosis (terror) while awaiting their cue. However, while the paper-bag method may be useful in helping with acute panic attacks, it is of no use to chronic overbreathers. It may temporarily restore normal blood gases, but it does nothing to correct the underlying cause: breathing-pattern disorders.

It is extremely dangerous during an acute asthma attack to try to control rapid, wheezy breathing using a paper bag. Increased drives to breathe are normal during an attack. It is on record that at least one person has breathed his last breath into a brown paper bag.

Recent medical research has revealed more about the physiological system derangements, metabolic imbalances, and anxiety-related symptoms caused by habitual over-breathing, but it is still an underrecognized and undertreated disorder.

Whether it is primarily a mental or a physical health problem has been hotly debated. Fortunately, the move towards holistic medicine, in which body and soul are treated together, has been of benefit to the vast number of people suffering from chronic hyperventilation and to their doctors, who can add this distressing disorder to their diagnostic repertoire.

I had a medical file as thick as a phone book, and I always seemed to be at the doctor's having tests for this and that. Nothing was ever found to be really wrong. But a doctor substituting for my GP nailed it straight away. My breathing was grossly askew, and my symptoms were a result of this. At last I had something to work on.

— Joan, 54

CHAPTER 2

Who Develops
Breathing-Pattern Disorders?

When I went to the physical therapist for breathing retraining, my
daughter went along and took her nine-year-old son—my grand-
son—who was off from school. It was really funny seeing how we
all breathed alike and had little habits the same. We all had disordered patterns—all three generations.

— Ann, 63

All sorts of people develop breathing-pattern disorders, and at
all ages. Note the following facts:

◆ Children are not exempt. Chronic blocked noses and
   habitual mouth-breathing often establish chaotic
   breathing patterns from quite early ages.

◆ People with asthma—about 14.9 million in the United
   States—are particularly prone to chronic hyperventilation. With recent advances in user-friendly inhalers
   to manage symptoms, few benefit from breathing
   retraining and physical therapies to improve respiratory function and the mechanical changes to the neck
   and chest muscles common in overbreathers.

◆ Following major surgery, some people find that
   the breathing techniques encouraged at the time of
   their operation—very big in-breaths to reexpand the
   lungs after anesthesia—trigger hyperventilation during

recovery. With the rapid turnaround in hospitals, or by having to travel to other centers for treatment, some do not receive postoperative care to correct this problem. (It's best to concentrate on restoring low, slow nose/abdominal breathing and relaxation between bouts of "big breathing" and coughing.)

◆ Those with more permanent lung damage—chronic obstructive airway diseases or emphysema, for instance—often develop inefficient breathing patterns, with HVS adding to their stress levels.

◆ People with heart disease and hypertension may also find that anxiety about health adds to their HVS symptoms. While medication to manage the disease is prescribed, often little attention is paid to the coexisting breathing disorder.

◆ Some women are extrasensitive to hormonal changes, either in the week before their period or in the second half of pregnancy. Higher progesterone levels increase respiratory drives. Carbon dioxide levels may be reduced by up to 25 percent, inducing HVS symptoms.

◆ Menopause, with its hormonal fluctuations, is also a common cause of breathing-pattern disorders.

◆ Older people facing retirement may have problems adjusting to aging, the loss of a loved one, or erratic health. They are prime candidates for breathing-pattern disorders.

◆ HVS is surprisingly common among teenagers, with raging hormones, peer pressures, parental expectations, and educational and recreational demands adding up to megastress.

♦ High achievers and workaholics who put huge pressures on themselves are sitting ducks for HVS. High stress levels equate with sympathetic-system overload.

♦ Victims of abuse or torture often suffer chronic breathing-pattern disorders and sympathetic-system overload, with a frightening array of symptoms adding to their distress.

♦ Migrant groups, adjusting to a new culture while grieving for the loss of their own, frequently have breathing-related disorders, especially if they are refugees from abuse or torture.

No one is immune, as the following accounts show:

Jane, 36

My first attack of acute hyperventilation happened at a street parade. It was hot, crowded, and noisy, and I left my husband and two kids to find some shade.

I couldn't stay still and paced up and down, feeling terrible. Then I lost my hearing and I felt dizzy, as though I might faint. But I didn't, and nothing seemed to change for about 15 minutes or so. I could see a policeman nearby, so I felt fairly safe.

I found my husband and got the keys to go back to the car. He could see I wasn't well so we went home. I went to my doctor the next morning. He took about 20 tubes of blood and did all kinds of tests, but they all came back negative. His diagnosis was that I had a virus—even though all the tests said I was in good health. I spent two weeks in bed, but after three weeks I still felt terrible so I abandoned the virus idea. I then went to another doctor for a second opinion and he diagnosed an anxiety disorder. He said it would go away, and no other help was offered. I didn't really know what to think about that diagnosis. I certainly *was* anxious about my symptoms, and I dreaded attacks.

I got heaps of self-help books—I had them stacked up by my bed. But I only looked at them; I couldn't actually do anything. I wasn't sleeping much by then, either. I was convinced I had a huge brain tumor that the doctors weren't telling me about. How could I continue to feel so spaced out and ill, yet have all my tests come back okay?

One evening not long after this I insisted on going to an accident and emergency clinic; I was about to die. There were around twenty people waiting, and I looked at all those sick people ahead of me. I couldn't wait for them. After all, they were only sick—I was dying! We raced into the pharmacy next door to ask the pharmacist to help me. He peered over his glasses and pigeonholed me instantly as a flake. He didn't think I was dying.

"I bet your house is tidy," he said. "You can come down and dust this place any time." He thought I was a rather extreme example of the worrywart, with a dash of over-achiever's zeal.

I begged for something to take that would at least help me to sleep. He suggested a strong over-the-counter sedative which would make me feel awful (he wasn't going to let me off lightly), but that I would sleep, and he said if that didn't work my husband should give me a good boxing round the ear. It was all very jokey, but no help at all to me or my husband.

I was getting frantic by now. Every scan, test, and X-ray showed I was well, but I still had symptoms—the dizziness, achy muscles (especially my upper chest, neck, and shoulders), terrible stomach upsets. I felt so unwell I had to give up my part-time job—a job I really loved. I didn't even want to go out.

I heard about HVS and went to a physical therapist to have that checked out. I hadn't been aware of my breathing except for the feeling I wasn't getting enough air—which I interpreted on an emotional level ("I'm going to die")—but I sighed all the time and hunched my shoulders up.

The physical therapist's lengthy assessment showed that my breathing rates and patterns were all over the place, and, mechanically, that my upper chest was doing all the work and I was holding myself tight around my waist—through all the anxiety and fear. I was mouth-breathing all the time, too. It felt really uncomfortable when I tried to nose-breathe. I was pushing truckloads more air through my chest than normal.

Going back over my history, it became apparent that the attack I had at the parade was a severe acute attack on top of what was probably long-standing chronic overbreathing. So what seemed normal after that dreadful episode wasn't normal at all. In fact, my resting breathing rate was twenty-four breaths a minute. (Normal is half that.)

We found, too, that things had been building up over many years, unnoticed or attributed to something else. My symptoms were worse premenstrually, and when I thought back to my pregnancies, I realized I probably had had undiagnosed postnatal depressions. Not long before the parade disaster, I'd been obliged to work full-time for a couple of months to cover for someone else—of course, I couldn't say no. And that had been one of the last straws on the camel's back. For a long time I'd been running on empty but had kept on going—just like everyone else. Hell, I was young and healthy.

Because I'd been in this spiral for so long, I was in such a mess that I agreed to have some counseling and to go on antianxiety medication that would relax my muscles and stop me from being on "red alert" all the time. I was very reluctant to take pills, but when I understood that the drug replaced stuff I wasn't producing enough of—serotonin—because of my stress, and that I needn't stay on them forever, I agreed. I hated it at first, but I stuck it out and after about 6 weeks it knocked the top off most of my anxieties.

It's given me space to work on the physical stuff—breathing properly again. Getting my physiology right and learning to relax, to let go—that's been unbelievably hard. Back to the beginning, really, as my physical therapist said. Just as it took me a long time to become unwell, it'll take time to become well. I have to be patient—and do the work.

Tom, 6

(As told by his mother.)

The school nurse called to say Tom was in the infirmary with stomach pains, and asked if I would come and pick him up. Even though he was the picture of health, he had been complaining of stomachaches prior to this, as well as other vague symptoms. He was happy at school and doing well. I thought he was breathing strangely, though (I'd read about breathing-pattern disorders in a magazine, so I was alert to a possible problem). He seemed to hunch his shoulders up and take big breaths into his upper chest through his mouth. I took him to our doctor for a checkup. She couldn't find anything wrong. I asked for a referral for physical therapy, which she reluctantly agreed to. I think she thought I was being too fussy.

During our first session, Tom was asked all sorts of questions, and what came out was truly bizarre. During physical education, Tom's teacher had told the boys that girls breathe with their stomachs and boys breathe with their upper chests. The manly look was to puff out your upper chest. He apparently singled Tom out as an example of "girl" breathing. The poor boy! He'd been struggling to be an upper-chest breather, but not only did it not feel right, it made him feel sick. He was so pleased to know "tummy breathing" was normal.

He had no problems getting back to "normal" breathing. And the physical therapist had an interesting conversation with his teacher!

Dan, 51

The first symptoms appeared in June last year. I was sailing with my wife, and there'd been storm warnings and the worries that go with that. (We were living on our boat.) One may assume that anxiety and apprehension were the cause of what happened next: erratic breathing, pain in the top of my head, and an overall feeling of exhaustion that lasted about an hour. My recovery was speedy once we got safely underway.

The next incident was in December, also on the boat, but in ideal conditions and in a nonstressful environment—a sudden feeling of dizziness, a pain in the head, and I semi-fainted. As quickly as it happened, I recovered. But a couple of hours later, getting out of the dinghy, my knees went wobbly and I had to slump back until I recovered a few minutes later. A doctor's appointment was made as a result of these frightening incidents, but after all sorts of tests nothing could be detected that may have caused the attacks. I was advised to take aspirin daily—the doctor thought blood clotting in the neck area may have been a factor.

In January I had further attacks, which my wife attributed to nerves, as there were some atrocious sailing conditions. Always afterwards there was a feeling of exhaustion.

Back home, my doctor thought I might have been having hyperventilation problems and booked me in for assessment with a breathing specialist.

Two days before my appointment, on the second day of a new job, I experienced another attack of breathlessness, dizziness, and disorientation. My whole body felt as though I were in an earthquake, but no one else could see this. I was driven to the hospital; following extensive tests, including several blood tests, it was revealed that my carbon dioxide levels were very, very low. When I had my appointment with the physical therapist, a breathing disorder was confirmed.

As a result of two visits, I have an awareness of the problem and the ability to deal with it. The problem has hardly arisen, and if it does, it can be countered easily.

For what it's worth, over the years I'd had a broken marriage, remarriage, problems with teenagers from two families that greatly affected me, early retirement from the police force due to burnout—all these were contributing factors. But what was so puzzling was that it was not until all these stresses were behind me and we were enjoying our new lifestyle that the symptoms appeared.

Fortunately, it was treated quickly.

Kate, 24

I'd been feeling a bit run-down, but I couldn't take a break. I'd just started my first job as a lawyer in a big law firm, and I was putting in a lot of extra time. Missed meals and late nights—I had a fairly active social life as well—took their toll.

I started feeling breathless running up stairs, and I found my workouts at the gym much harder than usual. People noticed I was sighing a lot too—not a good habit with clients.

I had other odd symptoms as well, like feeling light-headed, so I checked with my GP. I was anemic—I had a low red-blood-cell count. My doctor pointed out that red blood cells were the ones that carried the oxygen through the body. That's why I'd been feeling breathless—not enough oxygen carriers.

That was successfully treated, and I thought that'd be it—but I still had funny symptoms. It was a paramedic who told me I was hyperventilating, at a football match of all places. I checked on the Internet and found hundreds of references on the subject. It seems to be a widespread and common disorder. And even though I was no longer anemic, I was still over-breathing from habit. This was treated by physical therapy; I was only too keen to work on retraining my breathing back to normal. I'm symptom-free now.

Mary, 30

I was 24, recently married, and newly pregnant with my first baby. We had moved from one city to another and I really missed my family. I had a successful business—four florist shops, which meant a lot of early morning starts at the flower market and staff organization. There was a lot of pressure, which I managed well at first.

I worked right up until the day before my daughter was born, and it was a difficult birth. I was back at work 4 days later. The first business meeting I had to go to after this was when I had my first attack. I felt panic-stricken and I turned bright red, sweating and shaking. I had to leave the meeting. My fingers curled up and went stiff—it was terrifying.

My husband rushed me to the doctor. My blood pressure was up and my heart was racing. Because of concern about my blood pressure, my doctor sent me to be checked by a specialist. One thing is worse than high blood pressure, and that's worrying about it. I was very distressed.

The specialist shook my hand when we met and listened to my story. He said he knew exactly what was wrong with me just by shaking my hand (it was very clammy!). He also pointed out—my husband had noticed it too—that my breathing was fast and full of big sighs. He gave me a complete medical examination, more to put my mind at rest than anything else. Every test was normal. I felt very at ease and I trusted this man, but I felt so lousy that I knew there had to be something wrong with me.

He sent me for physical therapy to improve my breathing, as well as for counseling, but I had no one to help me get to my appointments—I hadn't built up a network of friends to help with my baby or other things. I was desperate to get to my appointments, but I missed them. I felt even more unwell, and helpless.

I did eventually get to a couple of appointments, but I still couldn't believe there wasn't something really wrong. I went back to the physician and he sent me off for a brain scan, just to reassure me. Over the next 5 years I had six brain scans—can you believe it?—all normal, of course. Plus every other test you can think of. I estimate that trying to find a diagnosis cost over $10,000.

I've had 5 years of slipping and sliding, but with counseling and regular respiratory-therapy checks, I've taken responsibility for my own wellness. I've made lifestyle changes to reduce stress. I take time for relaxation and time for exercise, and I no longer feel guilty about taking that time. I know my danger signs. I know what to do and why—and it works.

Jack, 62

I had a mild heart attack about 10 years ago, which gave me a fright. It made me give up smoking. I made a good recovery and was pretty well until a couple of years ago, when I started getting angina. Tests showed I had coronary artery disease, and I was scheduled for heart surgery, to have a triple bypass. It was very successful, and although I had a few breathing difficulties after the operation, I was up and about quickly and felt tremendous benefit. The exercises I had to do after the operation were designed to expand the lungs to prevent chest infections. I had this little gadget to encourage me to breathe in deeply. I got into the habit then of breathing in hard and using my upper chest.

A few months down the road I had sharp upper-chest pains, which worried me. But when I went for a checkup, my heart was fine. The cardiologist then sent me to a respiratory physician to check my lungs. They were okay too, but the way I was breathing was not. They diagnosed hyperventilation. My breathing rate was 26 a minute, and I was a mouth-breather. My wife had noticed this as well. When I put my hand on my breastbone, I could feel my upper chest working like bellows.

The chest doctor sent me for physical therapy, which I must say has been extremely helpful, not only in helping me get back to normal energy-efficient breathing, but also in sorting out the aches and pains in my chest and shoulders. I'm sleeping well again, and I garden and exercise with confidence.

CHAPTER 3

What Is "Good Breathing"?

My son reckons I'm contributing to global warming, the way I've been breathing. He's always on me about increased carbon dioxide emissions!

— Rob, 44

"Good breathing" means moving air in and out of the chest with the minimum of effort and using the chest muscles to their best advantage.

Three main groups of muscles are used for breathing.

The Diaphragm

Tailor-made for each person to supply the right amount of air to the lungs during rest and normal activity, this strong, thin, flat sheet of muscle is attached to the lower edges of the ribs. It separates the chest from the gut.

Shaped rather like the dome of an umbrella, it flattens down to expand the lungs. That's why your stomach expands as you breathe in. It draws in oxygen-rich air with very little effort. As the diaphragm relaxes, the dome shape is restored and carbon dioxide-rich air is gently exhaled. Diaphragmatic movement can vary from 1 centimeter at rest to 10 centimeters during exercise.

The diaphragm acts also as a vital pump, helping the heart to circulate blood up and down the body, and its gentle action on the stomach helps digestion as well as lymphatic flow.

Diaphragmatic, or abdominal, breathing is the most energy-efficient and relaxed way to breathe, and it helps reduce sympathetic tone (see the illustration of the autonomic nervous system on page 6).

Chest or Intercostal Muscles

These muscles join the ribs together and tighten to lift them, like a bird's wings, expanding the chest walls to draw in air and contracting back to push air out. They use about 20 percent more energy than the diaphragm.

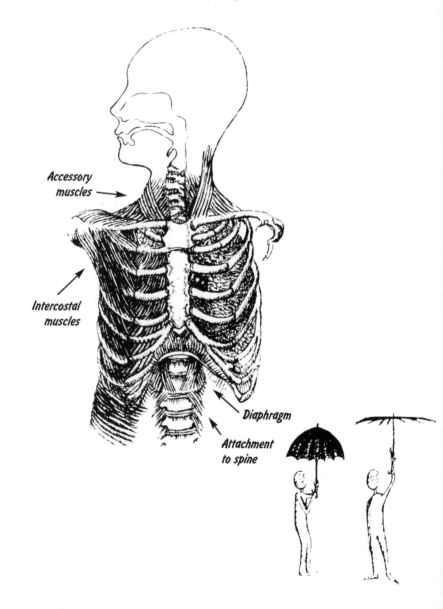

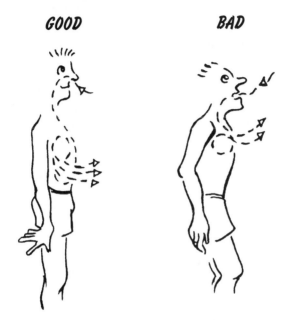

GOOD   BAD

In quiet breathing the lower ribs flare gently, helping the diaphragm, while the upper ribs remain relaxed. During moderate to strong exercise the upper chest opens up, like a reserve tank, to draw in extra oxygen-rich air; this also happens in response to fear or anger.

Accessory Muscles

The neck and shoulder muscles are used to tense and lift the upper chest in order to increase upper-chest volume; you can feel them working after strenuous exercise or effort. They work all the time in adults who have breathing rates of 20 or more a minute.

Stomach muscles are accessory muscles, too; you can feel them helping with breathing out during moderate to heavy exercise.

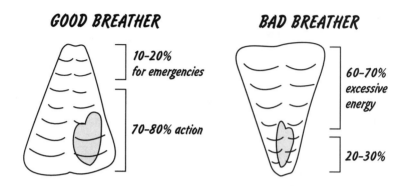

In normal, relaxed breathing, 70–80 percent of the work is done by the diaphragm, and the lower chest muscles do about 20–30 percent. The accessory muscles are on standby for extremes of effort or stress.

Habitual hyperventilators tend to reverse this ratio.

Oxygen and carbon dioxide levels, or blood gases, are kept in healthy balance by 12 regular breaths a minute (10–14 breaths is the normal range for adults). This moves 3 to 5 liters of air through the chest each minute.

Chronic overbreathers exchange up to double this amount of air. They are able to increase volumes by switching from nose-breathing to mouth-breathing. The next section explains why nose-breathing is important to respiratory health and the restoration of a normal energy-efficient breathing pattern.

Winning by a Nose... Jeff, 25

When I came to after having had surgery on my nose—which was injured playing football—I was in a blind panic. Both nostrils were packed with dressings and I felt I was suffocating. Breathing through my mouth felt so out of control and was making me feel very strange. My hands and lips were tingling. I rang the bell for help and the nurse was pretty abrupt with me. She said, "You're just hyperventilating," and virtually told me to get a grip and calm down. Boy, if she'd felt like I felt, she might have been a bit more helpful. Unfortunately, that experience stuck with me, and I had a lot of trouble with my breathing for a few months. I was as sick as a dog some days. Fortunately, my GP was on top of things and sent me to a physical therapist for some breathing retraining. It was quite an education, and I only needed one checkup after the first session. My breathing is good now.

One of the commonest findings in patients with breathing-pattern disorders is chronic mouth-breathing. Many have untreated nasal or sinus problems. The nose and nasal health have been woefully neglected in general medicine in recent times. Unless the person is sent to an ear, nose, and throat specialist for serious nasal problems, not much attention seems to be paid to the less dramatic but disturbing effects of chronic nasal-airflow problems—by either sufferer or doctor.

I talked to a pediatrician recently who honestly admitted that, as long as his asthmatic patients slept through the night and could go to school, he didn't bother much about their nasal stuffiness and resulting mouth-breathing patterns.

How the Nose Works

Our sense of smell is very important. It rests in the rhinencephalon, an area of the brain that developed early in our evolution and still has primitive connections to many other body systems that are vital to our survival.

While our noses have lost some of their finer "sniffing" abilities, they still have a vital role in guarding our respiratory health.

Watch a dog trotting round the neighborhood sniffing all the various "newsstands" on the way, gathering vast amounts of information about friends and foes. We probably get as much information reading the daily newspaper.

THE "SWEET" NOSE-BREATHER AND THE "BAD" MOUTH-BREATHER

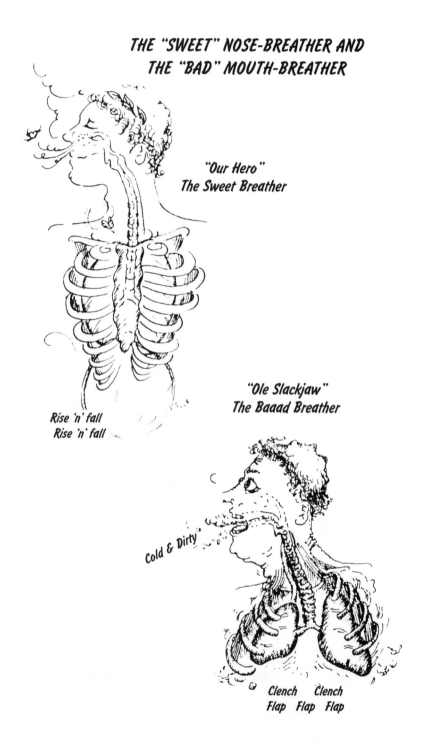

"Our Hero"
The Sweet Breather

"Ole Slackjaw"
The Baaad Breather

Rise 'n' fall
Rise 'n' fall

Cold & Dirty

Clench   Clench
Flap Flap Flap

The sense of smell is important to our emotional health, too—smell can trigger memories of good and bad environments, good and bad people, sad or happy times. It has links with many other vital body functions, such as the heart, the lungs, and the gut—through intriguing and complex reflexes and nerve connections.

The most obvious nasal reflex is the sneeze. The nasal linings coordinate with many other reflexes from the brain and spinal cord to produce a spontaneous "ah-choo" to clear irritants from the upper airways.

Body temperature is influenced by the temperature of the air breathed out of the nose. And think how powerful our nasal reflexes are in response to fumes. Very strong irritants can reduce or even stop breathing temporarily and affect the heart rate. Milder stimulants cause a reflex increase in breathing. This is why some people feel bad in shopping malls or airplanes: their symptoms are triggered by overbreathing in response to air fresheners or other fragrances pumped into air-conditioning systems.

Breathing through the nostrils draws air over fine, filtering hairs into the inner nose—then through turbinates, baffles, and nasal linings, swirling the air around so it is warmed and humidified in preparation for the lung.

Air breathed in through the mouth misses out on this "air-conditioning."

The nose has not only two external nostrils, but two inner noses, divided by the nasal septum, that work together. One dilates to carry the major part of the air stream, while the other rests, or clears out any debris. During waking hours these rhythmic cyclic changes happen every 2 to 4 hours. You can check this yourself by blocking one nostril to see which side is on duty.

When you're breathing through the nose, in normal health, there is roughly 50 percent more resistance to the airflow than with mouth-breathing. This becomes obvious when you switch from nose- to mouth-breathing—try it yourself.

This resistance creates pressure differences between the external nose and the lung, which are essential for efficient respiration.

It's interesting that this lowering of resistance was what Jeff found so distressing when he was forced to mouth-breathe after his nasal surgery. Fortunately, very few surgeons pack nostrils postoperatively.

Sleep and Nasal Congestion

If you sleep on your side, the lower nostril tends to congest while the upper nostril takes over. The head—and body—turn to reverse this pattern; these turning cycles are part of restful healthy sleep. The cycling rates vary with sleep patterns.

Sleeping in one position can lead to cramps, neck stiffness, backache, erratic breathing, and poor rest. Having too many turning cycles—thrashing about—is also unrestful. This is often caused by poor nasal and respiratory function during sleep, as anyone who has recently had a head cold will confirm.

Chronic snoring with interrupted breathing during sleep, combined with daytime sleepiness, needs further investigation. If you have this problem, you should discuss it with your doctor.

Long sequences of nights spent in unrefreshing sleep lead to a multitude of problems. Tension and anxiety, vivid dreams or nightmares, poor concentration, chronically disturbed breathing patterns—all these become part of feeling generally "stressed out."

Sleeping with the mouth closed can be hard. When you're really relaxed, the jaw relaxes too, with the mouth falling open. There's not much you can do about that, short of wearing a chinstrap like Monsieur Poirot, or taping your lips together as recommended by Buteyko practitioners. At least try going to sleep breathing through your nose. Don't worry if you wake with a dry mouth—as long as you slept well and wake refreshed.

Breathe Right-brand nasal strips, which stick to the outside of the nostrils, dilating them, can be of great benefit in getting used to nose-breathing at night.

Medical Treatments

When the nose becomes congested, the nasal sinuses (hollow areas in the supporting facial bones) become prime sites for inflammation and infection. Allergic reactions to inhaled irritants cause rhinitis or hay fever in susceptible people, also a trigger for chronic sinusitis; postnasal drip puts the lower airways and lungs at risk of infection. Mixtures of allergic reactions and chronic infections are common and can be very tricky to treat.

Nose-blowing, if too violent, can also cause sinus and ear problems. The best way to blow your nose and prevent damage to the tubes that connect with the inner ear is to block off one nostril while clearing the other *gently*. Teach your children by example.

Sorting out nasal and sinus problems takes a lot of detective work and patience. It's worth starting with a nasal scan if the problems are chronic. Only slightly more expensive than an X-ray, a nasal scan shows far more accurately the state of the nose and sinuses. You and your doctor can then be more specific with treatment options, rather than following the hit-and-miss approach of trying (and wasting) different sprays or drops in the blind hope they'll work.

If your doctor prescribes a nasal medication, make sure you know exactly what it's for, why you're taking it, and how to use it, and ask about and be prepared for any side effects. It is worth putting up with short-term discomfort for long-term relief.

Nasal medications fall into two groups, relievers and pre-venters:

◆ Relievers, in the short term, cause shrinkage of the nasal linings. They can be used intermittently, but mustn't be used continuously because overuse makes the nose clog up even more.

◆ Preventers have long-term anti-inflammatory and anti-allergic benefits. These are usually local steroids that coat the lining of the nose with minimal effect on the rest of the body. Commitment to regular use for long periods is essential to get the full benefit.

Both relievers and preventers come in drops, sprays, and aerosols. Sometimes it helps to change methods if one method seems ineffective.

Over-the-counter pills are useful for seasonal allergies. Antibiotics may be prescribed by your doctor to knock out bacterial infection (the full course of antibiotics must be taken).

Physical therapy offers ultrasound electrotherapy, pressure-point treatments, and acupuncture—worth a try if you'd pre-fer alternatives to drugs.

Alternative Remedies

There are also some old, inexpensive treatments that can be very effective in the early stages of infection.

Try steam inhalations with eucalyptus oil or Vicks VapoRub™. Talk to your pharmacist—some sell special steam-ers with shaped tops to direct the steam; these are safer for younger children, the very elderly, or those with disabilities to use than open bowls. Wear a shower cap to protect your hair.

Check out the natural foods store: there are many natur-opathic remedies that may work for you. They can be expen-sive, so ask for supporting literature.

Exercise is another treatment. The heel strike during running or brisk walking helps vibrate the sinus cavities. The nasal airways dilate, and circulation increases with aerobic exercise, helping sinus drainage.

Think about some of the external causes of nasal problems and how you can fix, change, or avoid them:

♦ allergies (pets sleeping on the bed, for instance)

♦ environmental pollution (smoky bars, dusty or dirty workplaces)

♦ mechanical obstruction (polyps or injury)

Think about the internal causes, too. With chronic breathing-pattern disorders, the breathing-control center in your brain wants to keep you overbreathing, and the mouth is the easiest route. Unfortunately, air is not warmed, filtered, or humidified when you mouth-breathe, whereas the nose is a built-in air conditioner.

Relearning nose-breathing can be very uncomfortable at first. Those who can't get the knack need to get help. Make an appointment with a physical therapist. Be kind to your lungs.

Nasal health is a top priority in restoring normal breathing patterns and better health and well-being—in the most surprising areas.

Nasal Wash

This recipe for nasal wash provides an easy, cheap, and effective remedy. Although salt is a preservative that will allow the concoction to last a while, you should make the solution fresh each day so as to avoid possible contamination.

Dissolve 1/2 teaspoon rock or sea salt and 1/2 teaspoon baking soda in 1 pint of hot, *boiled* water. (The salt helps reduce nasal-lining sogginess, and the baking soda acts like Teflon, preventing anything from sticking.) Fill a clean nasal-spray bottle and discard the excess solution.

Use the nasal wash morning and night: You can spray it into the nostrils using either a squeeze bottle or bulb syringe. If you do not have one of these devices or do not want to have to sterilize these objects on a daily basis, use the "snuffle" technique: After making the solution, wash your hands and dry them. Cupping one hand, pour about 1 tablespoon (½ oz.) into the palm of your hand and then, closing the other nostril, snuffle the saline into your nose. Repeat on the same side of the nose for a total of two handfuls of solution. Then clean the other nostril in the same fashion.

The most radical part of learning to nose-breathe again was that I could kiss properly. My boyfriend pointed out that kissing me used to be like kissing a gasping goldfish. And it's made the rest of my sex life so much better too, because I feel so much better. I hadn't realized what I was missing out on.

— Emma, 26

CHAPTER 4

Why Do People Become
Hyperventilators?

Someone recently pointed out that how many hours a week you work has almost become a status symbol. I and most of my contemporaries put in a 60-hour week, and I admit we do tend to boast about it. But the pressure I put myself under—it's killing me.

— *Dave, 37*

The respiratory center in the hindbrain responds to messages from different parts of the body, as well as from the higher brain or cerebral cortex. After a bout of rapid breathing, whether from hard exercise, high emotions, or danger, the respiratory system gradually allows the breathing rate to slow down as the body regains balanced blood gases.

In those under prolonged stress, the respiratory center adapts gradually to accept lower or fluctuating carbon dioxide levels and respiratory alkalosis. Various parts of the body and mind may feel extremely uncomfortable with the blood gas imbalances, but the respiratory center rides roughshod over any distress signals it receives; it keeps instructing the lungs to breathe hard and fast.

The causes for this may be mechanical, starting after chest surgery or in lung diseases that cause airflow disturbances, for example, bronchiectasis and tuberculosis. The disorder may start after physical illnesses such as pneumonia, chest infections, glandular fever, and viral infections.

In addition, HVS often appears during or after emotional upheavals such as the following:

♦ death of a spouse, lover, or relative

♦ separation or divorce

♦ losing a job

♦ change in status, growing up, aging

♦ moving to a different town

♦ living in a war zone

Exercise, too, may trigger hyperventilation attacks when stress levels are high and fitness levels are low.

What Does It Feel Like to Hyperventilate?

The most common phrases hyperventilators use are:

♦ "I thought I was going to pass out—I couldn't seem to take the next breath in."

♦ "I never seem to get a satisfying breath."

♦ "I've never been quite the same since my operation." (Or accident, or breakup...)

♦ "I really thought I was losing my mind."

♦ "I thought I was dying."

In sudden attacks, people are usually less aware of heaving upper-chest breathing but are all too aware of the anxiety and strange symptoms that might follow, such as dizziness, tingling fingers and lips, and panicky thoughts.

Those who rush to their doctor may be prescribed a mild tranquilizer after a full checkup and given a reassurance that "nothing's wrong." For some this is enough to break the cycle.

But others who find their strange and frightening symptoms recurring are left to imagine the worst.

Heart attack! Brain tumor! Colon cancer!

Do they go back to their doctor or write their will?

Once the breathing pattern becomes centered in the upper chest and away from the diaphragm, more widespread and frightening symptoms begin to emerge, and a Catch-22 cycle is established.

Is Hyperventilation Syndrome Very Common?

The short answer is yes.

One group of European researchers described HVS as a "silent epidemic." An American source claims that 6–11 percent of the general patient population suffers from HVS, with between two and seven female sufferers (ages 15 to 55) for every male. British figures are even higher, suggesting that up to 40 percent of patients sitting in doctors' waiting rooms have disordered breathing patterns. All specialists (cardiologists, gastroenterologists, neurologists, rheumatologists, etc.) attract high numbers, too, with an estimated 50–70 percent of patients habitually overbreathing.

The Hazards of Heavy Breathing

♦ Habitual mouth-breathers develop irritable upper airways, with the risk of repeated upper respiratory tract infections. A very common sign of hyperventilation is repeated throat clearing: the a-hrrrrrm bug.

- Chronic overbreathing triggers increased histamine levels in the blood. Sweaty palms and flushed cheeks are signs of this. Those with allergies—and this includes people with asthma, hay fever, food intolerances, and skin rashes—find their symptoms get worse.

- Response to pain is amplified, with stiffness, aching, and tension in muscles, tendons, and joints resulting from chronic hyperventilating and poor metabolism.

- Heart-disease-type symptoms, such as chest-wall tightness or pain and palpitations, can be downright terrifying.

- Mental fuzziness, headaches, or memory lapses erode self-confidence, especially if work suffers.

- Making love can become a nightmare—for both partners—if the heavy breathing needed to reach orgasm leads to a panic attack.

- Vivid or bad dreams and disturbed sleep patterns often accompany hyperventilation, making for round-the-clock distress and exhaustion.

Almost every system in the body suffers. Fear of the relentless symptoms drives the respiratory center into top gear, and the cycle is complete. Hyperventilation syndrome gives free rein to the fear... and the symptoms... and to the bewilderment of sufferer, family, and friends.

It was a mystery to me how Susie, once so outgoing and full of energy, had turned into a fearful, tired shadow of her old self. I admit I wasn't very sympathetic. It was tough on our kids. I had no idea what to do or who to turn to.

— *Edward, 40*

CHAPTER 5

What Can I Do About HVS?

Within 2 months I'd been to the emergency room six times with chest pains and breathing very fast. I had pins and needles and felt sick each time. I had lots of different tests and nothing was wrong. This last time a doctor I hadn't seen before immediately diagnosed hyperventilation and sent me off for physical therapy.

— Mele, 42

As yet there is no reliable repeatable laboratory test to confirm a diagnosis of HVS, but after a thorough checkup to rule out organic disease, your doctor may check for HVS in several ways.

The doctor may use skilled observation to detect irregular or fast breathing patterns or signs of sympathetic-system overload (rapid pulse, sweating, jumpiness).

You may be asked to do the "think test," in which breathing patterns are monitored as you talk about symptoms and anxieties. Most people can pinpoint a stressful event that, when brought to mind, triggers most of their symptoms, along with increased breathing rates or sighing.

You might be asked to take the 12-breath test, an exercise in voluntary overbreathing. To many sufferers' amazement this can reproduce exactly their distressing symptoms. It is more useful as a teaching tool than as an accurate diagnostic test.

There are three main types of chest pain associated with hyperventilation syndrome:

♦ Sharp pains felt while breathing in, often just below the left breast, from pressure on the diaphragm due to a bloated stomach, filled by "air-gulping" and causing spasm of the diaphragm and pain.

♦ Dull, aching chest-wall soreness, often felt after exercise; this is due to overstretching of the chest-wall (intercostal) and accessory muscles, or from the heart itself banging on the inside of the chest wall.

♦ Heavy pain behind the breastbone radiating to the neck and arms; this happens when the blood supply to the heart muscle itself is reduced in response to altered blood chemistry from chronic overbreathing, with spasming of the coronary arteries.

Unfortunately, all three types of pain are difficult to reproduce on demand; the multiple stressors (physical, social, and emotional) that combine with hyperventilating to bring on chest pain are not found in the security of your doctor's rooms.

Other, more high-tech methods of diagnosis are available, but because blood-gas levels fluctuate in chronic hyperventilators, it may be difficult to pick up the problem from a single test. More often than not, it's a matter of ruling out what it *isn't*.

Unfortunately, for your doctor to test you for hyperventilation, he or she needs to be aware of the disabling effect of the condition. It may be reassuring to be told, "Go away, you're in great health," but only until the symptoms materialize again; when they do, often they seem much worse. If no one believes your symptoms are real, does it mean it's all in your mind? Or, worse still, incurable?

People who already have asthma, heart disease, or chronic pain symptoms may be made worse by erratic overbreathing. Often, instead of recognizing hyperventilation, their doctors load them with extra drugs for the existing condition. This is hardly surprising since medical training has in recent years offered only passing mention of the subject of hyperventilation—usually just the acute phase. This results in a focus only on symptoms.

Doctors often treat the individual symptoms of HVS, not the underlying disorder causing all the distress. It's rather like prescribing skin lotion to someone with yellow jaundice.

Where to Start?

One doctor described hyperventilation syndrome as "a diagnosis begging for recognition." Once it has been diagnosed, though, there are a number of possible treatments that your doctor may offer.

Drug Options

The most common drugs prescribed are tranquilizers, which may be lifesavers in the short term but leave the habitual overbreathing component untreated. Long-term use of tranquilizers exposes you to the added risks of dependency and addiction—and a greater loss of self-reliance.

Antidepressants that are physically nonaddictive are worth considering when disabling anxiety, fearfulness, or phobias exist. They can be seen as a "chemical holiday," rebuilding levels of serotonin (a mood enhancer) worn down by stress. They can provide shelter from the storm: room to restore normal breathing patterns and develop an effective relaxation response.

Physical Coping Skills

Long-term "bad breathers" benefit from physical therapy sessions both for breathing retraining and for sorting out the complex physical side effects that radiate from HVS and its symptoms. Musculoskeletal problems commonly add to the mix and need special attention.

Upper-chest breathing requires sustained effort from accessory muscles, which were primarily designed for a supporting role only. Physical symptoms such as headaches, costochondritis (painful rib joints), and neck and shoulder stiffness and pain often result, adding to the general misery. Motor patterns change, making the upper chest muscles the dominant muscles of breathing, instead of the diaphragm.

Mental Coping Skills

Some chronic hyperventilators develop avoidance behaviors in an attempt to control symptoms by controlling their environment. Perpetual anxiety about maintaining control is a common cause of phobias. The most common of these are:

♦ fear of being away from home (agoraphobia)

♦ fear of enclosed spaces (claustrophobia)

♦ fear of travel, either driving or flying

Anxiety about sex may also lead to avoidance through fear of symptoms, fear of failure, or fear of not being able to cope with intense emotion.

Expert psychiatric or psychological help would be advisable if these problems continue.

The BETTER Breathing Plan

The options listed above do not provide the whole answer, although they are a valid and vital part of treatment.

There is another treatment, one that is simple, although it requires—like most things—commitment to change. The six-step plan detailed in the next part of the book uses the letters BETTER to cover important aspects of recovery.

B	**Breathing retraining**
E	**Esteem**
T	**Total body relaxation**
T	**Talk**
E	**Exercise**
R	**Rest and sleep**

Read on to discover how to combat HVS and restore normal breathing (and blood gases) and to look at ways to cope with the pressures causing these problems. Use the charts at the back of the book to monitor your progress. And "when in doubt, breathe out."

This breathing business has to do with shedding some of the clutter that constricts us as tightly as our grandmothers' corsets. It's about embracing a sense of something special, easily and immediately accessible right there inside us, like an echo from childhood.

— *Pru, 55*

PART II

The BETTER Breathing Plan

CHAPTER 6

The BETTER Breathing Plan: B—Breathing Retraining

The most crucial step was to start a daily practice. No big deal—just 5 minutes of breathing down into my belly, concentrating on the exhale, embracing the stillness before the inhale. It was ridiculously hard at first. Then it became as effortless and essential as a morning pee. Five minutes soon slipped into 10 then 20 minutes.

— Jenny, 54

For people with chronic hyperventilation and disordered breathing patterns, restoring a normal breathing pattern takes a great deal of patience and concentration, as well as regular practice. Some are able to switch easily back to normal breathing, while others may take months, sometimes up to a year, to be free of symptoms. It may be uncomfortable at first, but using conscious effort to restore your natural unconscious pattern enables the respiratory control centers in your brain to reset from overdrive back to normal.

The following simple techniques will help turn you into a good breather, although you may need extra help. A session with a physical therapist is a good way to check out any musculoskeletal or postural problems that may have developed and to cover coping strategies for stress and tension. It's much easier to learn from a hands-on assessment.

The four basic steps in breathing retraining are:

♦ becoming aware of faulty breathing patterns

♦ learning low, slow nose-breathing

♦ learning to relax the upper chest and shoulders

♦ restoring normal breathing volumes and rates (10–14 breaths per minute)

Big Breaths Versus Deep Breaths

From a very early age, often at school, people learn to stick out their chests and suck in their stomachs like soldiers or "Baywatch" stars. Ask anyone to take a deep breath, and chances are he'll fill up his whole chest and take a *big* breath instead.

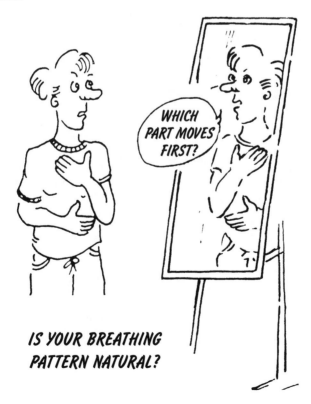

Try it. Stand in front of a mirror and place the hand you write with on your stomach between your lower ribs and navel. Then put the other hand on your breastbone, just below your collarbone.

Take a deep breath and observe three things.

- ◆ Which part of your chest moved first?

- ◆ Which part of your chest moved most?

- ◆ Did you breathe in through your nose or mouth?

If you breathed in through your nose, your stomach expanded first, and you felt minimal upper-chest movement, then you executed a true deep breath, reflecting a natural breathing pattern.

If you breathed in fast through your mouth, you could see and feel your upper chest heave first, and you felt little or no stomach movement or drew it *in*, then you might have a disordered breathing pattern.

Strategies for Breathing Retraining

It's best to start out by practicing while lying comfortably on your back. This means you can switch off all your postural reflexes and relax your whole body while you retrain. Most people agree it's easier to focus on abdominal breathing this way while relearning the natural pattern. Getting the knack of abdominal breathing while lying down makes the progression to doing so while sitting and standing easier.

Lying with a pillow under your head and knees, concentrate on the out-breath. You may find it easier at first to lie with your hands clasped behind your head, to relax the upper-chest muscles. Let the air "fall" out of your chest without pushing. Breathe in gently through your nose and let go right away, concentrating on breathing out lightly. Shoulder and upper chest relaxation is vital.

With lips together and jaw loose, draw air lightly in through your nose, relaxing and expanding your waist, feeling your stomach puff up. Let go right away and allow the elastic recoil of your diaphragm and lower chest to breathe air out effortlessly and quietly.

If you feel dizzy, it means you're still big-breathing rather than deep-breathing. Cup both hands over your mouth and nose and rebreathe carbon dioxide-rich air for five or six breaths, then rest. Repeat this until the dizziness has gone.

Start with very light, small abdominal breaths. Make sure you let go right away at the top of the in-breath—don't hold—and that you relax at the end of the out-breath. If you feel like taking in huge drafts of air, resist the temptation. Remember: If you breathe in big, you're going to breathe out big too, further depleting carbon dioxide levels.

Silently repeat to yourself, "Lips together, jaw relaxed, breathing low and slow." This mental chant helps concentration.

Imagine a piece of fine elastic around your waist, stretching as you inhale. Or think of breathing into your (loose) belt or waistband. Check chest movements with your hands.

Spend at least 10 minutes per session. Repetition is essential.

Timing

Once you feel confident about your breathing pattern, concentrate on the rate.

Time yourself by watching the second hand on a watch or clock for half a minute while you count your breaths (breathing in and out is one breath). Aim to breathe about twelve breaths per minute—six per half minute.

NORMAL AND ABNORMAL BREATHING PATTERNS

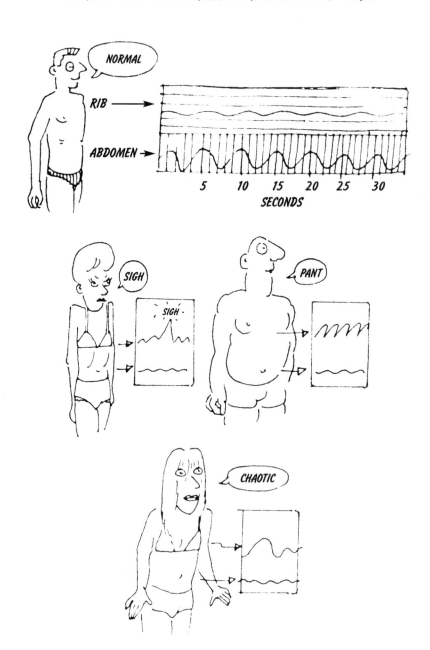

If you are breathing much faster than that, relax, let go, and check again in a couple of minutes. If you are too much slower, lighten your breathing—and relax.

The relaxed pause at the end of exhalation means breathing out takes longer than breathing in. One imaginative man found that, instead of counting, it helped his timing to mentally say the words "Bombay" (breathe in), "Sapphire" (breathe out), and "Gin" (relax)!

Exhalation may be more prolonged (Sapp-h-i-r-e) in people with chest disorders such as asthma or chronic obstructive respiratory diseases. This is normal.

Keeping Up the Practice

Practice the new low, slow breathing pattern lying on your side, sitting, and standing. When you walk or go up or down stairs, synchronize your breathing with movement. For example, breathe in for two steps, out for three.

At first, if you've been addicted to mouth/upper-chest breathing, nose/abdominal breathing will feel peculiar. Some describe it as "back to front" breathing. Others report uncomfortable feelings of air hunger. This is a good sign, showing you are making progress. Your respiratory center is being challenged to accept normal carbon dioxide levels; it will try to make you "big-breathe" again.

When you feel breathless

STOP—check your chest

DROP—relax shoulders and upper chest

FLOP—relax all over

Use rest positions (see the illustrations on page 52) whenever and wherever you get short of breath. Focus on low, slow nose-breathing.

It may take a long time and a great deal of practice to get your diaphragm strong and working confidently and for your respiratory center to accept normal blood-gas levels again. Don't be hard on yourself if you slip back into erratic patterns. Just concentrate on the next breath and getting it right.

REST POSITIONS

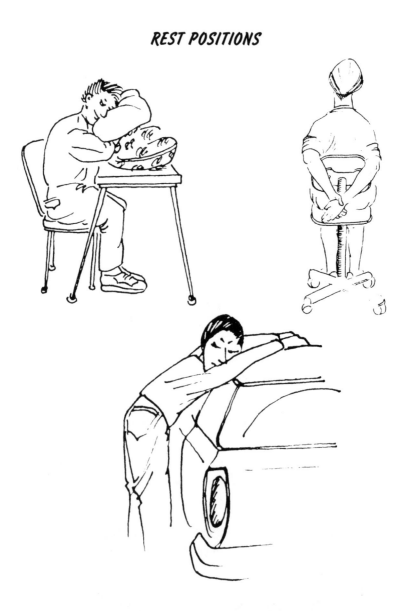

Set the alarm 5 minutes early, and every morning, before you get out of bed, lie on your back for a few minutes, practicing low, slow, relaxed breathing. Establish the pattern for the day.

For the first week of retraining, schedule two 10-minute sessions in the lying-down position each day, morning and evening. Reduce to once a day in week 2. Step up to twice a day again after bad days or stressful times.

During the day, every hour on the hour, check your chest, correct your breathing, and then *forget it.* Regular repetition is the best way to reinforce healthy breathing patterns—but don't be obsessive.

In bed at night, repeat the morning breathing routine, lying on your left side to help you go to sleep.

As you become reaccustomed to breathing properly, there will be less need to check the chest often. During stressful times, however, it pays to check breathing rates and patterns. Concentrating on this physical aspect helps dampen anxieties.

Common Mistakes and Problems

♦ Your diaphragm may be a bit jumpy at first, especially if it has been out of action for a while. Like any other group of muscles that have been out of use, your diaphragm may need strengthening.

If you find yourself breathing in a jerky "staircase" fashion, mildly resisted breathing helps. A 5-pound sack of flour—or a pumpkin or watermelon—placed just below the navel while lying down is ideal. (One woman found that her iron made a perfect weight.) If you have problems with gastric reflux (heartburn), practice in a semi-reclining position.

♦ Those on steroids, such as prednisone, need to pay special attention to maintaining diaphragm strength. Loss of condition in larger muscle groups, for example,

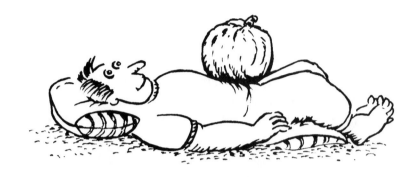

thigh muscles, is a common side effect of steroid use, and they can weaken the diaphragm, too. Strengthening exercises restore muscle power. Talk to your physical therapist.

♦ Those with asthma—both children and adults—need to pay special attention to their breathing after a bout of wheezing. Breathing may be chaotic during an attack, switching from upper to lower chest with little chance of control; this is normal—an increased respiratory drive is natural at this time.

Using rest positions and the "stop, drop, flop" routine helps combat the stress and fear while waiting for the asthma medications to work. Once the attack is over, reestablishing low-volume nose-breathing and relaxing the upper chest must be top priority.

♦ Your body will play all sorts of tricks to start you over-breathing again. The urge to sigh, yawn, or gulp air will seem overwhelming at times, and very uncomfortable at first. Remember, this is a sign of progress: your respiratory centers are frantically trying to make you hyperventilate again. With regular and determined practice, your respiratory centers will adjust to accept a balanced pH and normal ventilation.

To resist the urge to overbreathe, try swallowing hard and continue breathing low and slow.

♦ Wearing tight-fitting clothes and belts restricts normal breathing. Loosen up. Wear suspenders or elasticized belts.

♦ During heavy exercise, although it's normal to mouth-breathe in order to inhale extra oxygen, don't forget to resume nose-breathing as soon as you can after you are finished.

♦ Another popular mistake is to "brace" or fill up the upper chest, holding in huge volumes of air while using the diaphragm to breathe in more. Breathing this way makes symptoms worse.

It is just as important to relax the upper chest and shoulders as it is to breathe low/slow/through the nose.

A relaxing image to use while focusing on low, slow nose-breathing is to imagine breathing in through your heels.

When you feel your breathing is high in your chest, remember to:

♦ relax your shoulders by using a rest position (see page 52);

♦ keep lips together, jaw relaxed, shoulders dropped;

♦ concentrate on low, slow nose-breathing until you feel calm.

In other words, stop, drop, flop.

I've changed my life by changing the way I breathe. It feels dramatic, a magical shift for me. Nothing looks different from the outside—it's just that every day I feel lighter, at ease.

— Jenny, 54

CHAPTER 7

The BETTER Breathing Plan: E—Esteem

Looking through some photos of about 5 or 6 years ago, I was struck by how confident and "together" I looked then. Remembering those times made me realize how down I was now, and how timid I'd become—never sure if I was going to be okay or not in different situations. A recent photo showed me with my shoulders nearly up to my ears and looking pretty glum. I really had lost a lot of confidence in myself.

— Peter, 31

Most chronic hyperventilators suffer from a battered self-image. Good days may be few and far between, and these are overshadowed by the fear and loathing of bad days. Gradual erosion of confidence—feeling you are letting yourself or your friends down—adds to the general lack of self-worth. Strong positive emotions such as love, happiness, and laughter gradually get pushed aside by anxiety, anger (often repressed), and depression.

While you might receive support during times of major personal upheaval, little attention is paid to the cumulative effects of minor everyday hassles.

If left unresolved, these can build up to major proportions. The skill of being able to say, "Sorry, but no" to demands you know will overload you is a very important one to master.

The Power of Laughter

Loosening up, relaxing, and finding some humor in your life will prove that laughter is a powerful chemical-free remedy. Laughter benefits the whole person, body and soul; a good belly laugh liberates the mind from repetitive, often negative, thought patterns.

One group of researchers found that increased levels of immunoglobulins (antibodies) were produced in people watching funny films over those watching dreary ones. Laughter also seems to reduce the output of the stress hormone adrenaline, and just as exercise releases opioid peptides (hormones that make you feel good, such as endorphins), so does laughter. The final bonus is the exquisite relaxation that follows laughter and enjoyment.

Use of Language

Breaking the *tension* ➔ *HVS* ➔ *anxiety* ➔ *HVS* cycle requires a firm commitment to a change in outlook as well as in breathing patterns. Language and choice of words play an important role. To start with, eliminate the words "should," "if only," and "what if" from your vocabulary.

Being aware of negative or illogical thought and speech patterns helps you to change them. Listen to yourself. If you catch yourself thinking, "I'll never be able to manage..." or "I'm always letting people down...," gently question yourself. Always? Never? Think about it.

Depression

Fear of losing control is especially strong in chronic hyperventilators. This often leads to repression of normal emotions and the withholding of love, warmth, anger, or sadness.

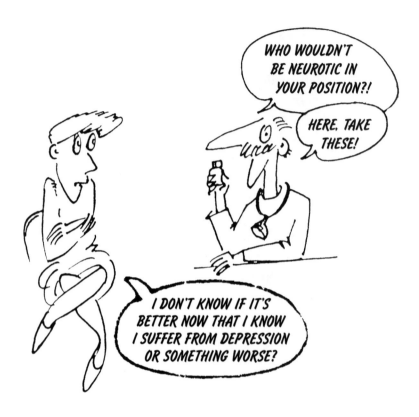

Unexpressed grief, fear, or resentment puts you in the fast lane to depression and withdrawal from everyday knockabout life.

At the risk of giving depression a good name, it is a fairly normal reaction to prolonged bouts of symptomatic hyperventilation. If there is nothing obvious to have surgically removed or to take a pill for, anxiety and depression are reasonable enough reactions to feeling constantly off-key. Treating the symptoms with drugs without paying attention to the breathing disorder is going to be of limited value to the sufferer and of great expense to our already overburdened health-care system.

More sinister, though, with the accompanying wearing away of self-esteem comes the likelihood of turning hyperventilators into chronic invalids. If the patient is shunted from specialist to specialist trying to find a diagnosis, undergoing all sorts of invasive or risky investigations with no relief, it's not surprising anxiety and depression become chronic.

Stress

Stress is essential to life—we'd be dead without it. But too much stress can lead to our ending up dead, as well.

One thing we can consciously control when managing stress responses is our breathing, which has a direct and indirect effect on the way we react. On the other hand, once your nervous system starts signaling "Stress attack!," abusing stimulants (coffee, cigarettes, alcohol, or recreational drugs) to boost flagging energy levels is asking for trouble.

Good ways to prevent overreaction to stressors include:

◆ accepting that it's how we respond to stress, not the stress itself, that does the damage

◆ realizing that breathing in excess of metabolic need affects all our body systems

◆ understanding that breathing, while mostly automatic, is also under conscious control

◆ using breathing techniques to help us avoid body-chemistry imbalances and the symptoms caused by overbreathing

Restoring a strong and healthy self-image means you're more likely to take notice of your body's reactions to stress, tiredness, and the early signs of exhaustion.

Think about lifestyle changes to reduce stress levels. Schedule time for breathing retraining, relaxation, massage, exercise, and sleep to absorb the effects of stress.

Body Mechanics and Posture

Good posture is a very important ingredient in combating HVS.

Check regularly: imagine being suspended by a fine thread from the back of the top of your head. Stretch up tall to prevent breaking this phantom thread.

Always sit with your bottom snug against the back of the chair. Maintaining good posture while sitting prevents your upper spine from sagging and compressing your lower chest and gut. Apart from the mechanical advantages to the process of breathing itself, holding and carrying yourself well—standing or sitting—makes you appear confident to others.

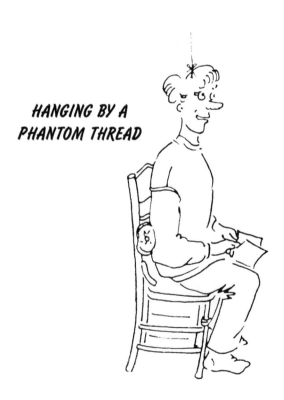

HANGING BY A PHANTOM THREAD

Tell a Friend

A potent way of taking the fear out of HVS is to tell *five* people whom you know about it. Explain the symptoms, how they start, and how you handle them. You'll be surprised how many other people have experienced it.

Unraveling the tight spiral of HVS can be a long yet illuminating process. However, gaining insight into the mechanisms that bring on HVS is only the starting point. Dealing with its effects may require extra assistance. If you need it, plenty of help exists out in the community to rebuild a healthy self-image.

Family, individual, and group counseling are available from a variety of agencies. Check with your local library for information. Browse through the dozens of excellent self-help books on the shelves. Or call your local United Way office for advice.

Coming to grips with HVS, and getting it off your chest, will put you back in the driver's seat and in—not under or out of—control.

When it was pointed out to me, I saw it was so true. I used negative language against myself nearly all the time. On top of that I seemed to sigh every time I finished saying anything. Especially after being on the phone. It was such a habit!

— Rose, 41

CHAPTER 8

The BETTER Breathing Plan: T—Total Body Relaxation

I felt very restless and uncomfortable even thinking about my breathing. When I lay on my back, I felt incredibly tense. Then I was asked to clasp my hands behind my head. It was amazing, because immediately I could feel my lower chest and diaphragm area working properly, without even trying. Soon I felt intensely relaxed—I actually started to laugh, I felt so good. It wasn't nervous laughter—just a fantastic letting go.

— Peter, 31

If you've been struggling for weeks, months, or even years with chronic hyperventilation, bizarre symptoms, fear, and tension, you may find it extremely hard to let go and relax. Releasing physical tension helps release mental tension, but the negative, repetitive thoughts that spin in your mind like hamsters running on a wheel may be just as hard to subdue as trigger-happy lungs.

Learning the knack of switching on relaxation when familiar hyperventilation symptoms reappear—and they will in times of stress—is an effective way of stopping symptoms in their tracks. It's difficult at first to feel you can release tension or to feel you can take time out to practice relaxation techniques. But daily dips into the relaxation response pay off, giving you more reserves to cope with the daily pressures—good and bad—that are part of normal life.

Remember that all relaxation methods start with low, slow nose-breathing, so mastering the techniques set forth in Chapter 6 is essential before continuing further.

Choosing a Suitable Relaxation Method

There are plenty of methods to choose from. Your choice will depend on whether mental or physical tension is more of a problem and where you are at the time. Knowing a variety of methods helps you be more adaptable.

Most physical and respiratory therapy clinics teach various types of relaxation as part of general stress management. Check with your doctor.

The Hyperventilator's Special

Relaxing in a prone position is ideal for hyperventilators. This involves lying on the belly and especially suits people who feel vulnerable or ill at ease lying on their backs. Lying facedown has a built-in sense of safety, with the soft underbelly protected by the spine.

The main elements of relaxation can be practiced. These include:

♦ abdominal breathing

♦ switching off antigravity or postural reflexes

LYING IN A PRONE POSITION

♦ arousing awareness of tension

♦ reducing sympathetic system tone (your body's stress response)

Preparation

Schedule a time—at least 10–15 minutes at first. Mark time out for relaxation breaks in your day planner or daily chores list.

Choose a quiet place to practice and take the phone off the hook or turn down the ring volume. Tell those around you what you are doing and why, and ask not to be disturbed. Even quite young children can be cooperative about "your time" and may even enjoy timekeeping.

Technique

Lying face down on a bed, put a firm pillow under your hips to free the diaphragm and another under your ankles to relax the back. You may need a soft pillow under your upper chest if you have a stiff neck.

If you can lie with your arms up, hands under your forehead, this helps suppress upper-chest breathing, as in the forward-leaning rest position (see page 52). If this makes your shoulders uncomfortable, keep your arms by your sides.

Don't go to sleep in this position if you have restricted neck movement.

You can practice some mental relaxation techniques (see pages 66 to 70) or listen to soothing music. After initial concentration on breathing low and slow for three or four breaths, forget about breathing...and...let go.

Relaxing this way is surprisingly rejuvenating.

Progressive Muscle Relaxation

This involves methodically stretching muscle groups for 5 or 6 seconds and then letting go for 10–15 seconds, concentrating on the difference between tension and release. It is an excellent way of pinpointing tension zones, such as your neck, scalp, shoulders, hands, and lower back. Most people doing this relaxation technique for the first time are surprised at the amount of physical strain they've been holding on to, and even more surprised at how good it feels to let it go.

The whole process takes 10–15 minutes at first. But if you practice regularly, you'll find it takes less and less time to switch off, and you can continue with "mini-relaxes." This technique is easy to learn and can be adapted to doing while sitting in a chair, at work, or on planes, buses, or trains.

Technique

1. Lie on your back, put a pillow under your head and another under your knees, and cover up with a blanket. Begin with two or three slow, light abdominal breaths, then forget your breathing.

2. Starting with your left leg, pull your toes up towards you, pressing the back of your knee into the pillow and tightening your whole leg to the hip (your heel will lift). Hold for five seconds—and let go slowly, relaxing for 10–15 seconds. Repeat with the right leg.

3. Continue, using the same timing, as you stretch and elongate the fingers and thumb of your left hand. Let go slowly... relax. Repeat, using the right hand.

4. Push your left elbow gently into the bed. Let go slowly... relax. Repeat with the right elbow.

5. Slide your hands down the bed towards your feet, feeling the stretch to your shoulders and neck. Let go slowly... relax.

6. Tuck in your chin and gently press your head back into the pillow, stretching the long muscles up the back of your neck. Let go slowly... relax.

7. Very lightly bring your teeth together. With lips closed, separate your teeth a little and move your jaw slightly from side to side. Stop. Swallow hard...and relax, with your tongue resting on the floor of your mouth.

8. Screw up your nose. Let go...relax.

9. Think of your eyelids as being light as feathers resting softly over your eyes. With eyes remaining closed, raise your eyebrows as high as you can...and let go slowly, feeling your brow and scalp smooth and relax. This is a common area of tension. Repeat two or three times.

10. Check for tension zones and repeat the sequences in those areas that still feel tight. At first you may have to repeat the tensing/relaxing routine ten or more times before you feel release.

11. When you feel you have unwound, rest and enjoy the feeling. Keep nagging or disruptive thoughts at bay by focusing on neutral repetitive ones, for example, mentally chanting the multiplication table.

Mental Relaxation Methods

There are many of these, but I will give details here only of the easiest. Look in your local library for relevant books and tapes. Make relaxation as important and regular as cleaning your teeth.

Passive Mental Relaxation

This involves sitting comfortably, eyes closed, hands on thighs, palms turned up.

Start with abdominal breathing. After three or four breaths, stop concentrating on breathing or on trying to relax, but passively accept whatever floats through the mind. Focus

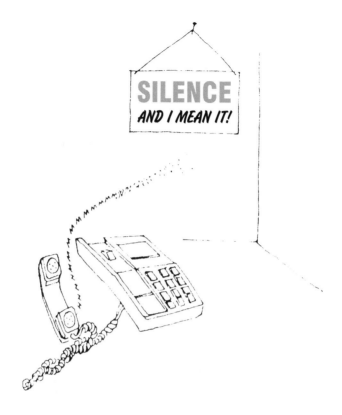

your concentration by silent repetition of a short word (try repeating the word "one" with each breath out).

Along with mental relaxation, you will experience deep physical relaxation.

Transcendental Meditation

Introduced to the West over 30 years ago, transcendental meditation (TM) is still a popular relaxation and meditation method. It's a type of passive mental relaxation, wherein an individual word is rapidly and silently repeated while focusing on deep physical and mental relaxation for 20 minutes twice a day. Nagging conscious thoughts are pushed out by the silent repetition of your given word.

Most major towns have a TM center. Joining a TM center is relatively expensive, but for people who have difficulty getting started with relaxation, the group support is helpful.

Autohypnosis

This method involves sitting fully supported in a chair about three yards from a wall, focusing on a spot on the wall just above eye level.

Counting breaths backward from 100, picture yourself floating and free. As your eyes start to feel heavy, let them close, and stop counting when you feel floppy and pleasantly relaxed. You will be fully awake and aware of your surroundings, and as soon as you want to finish, count three breaths to slowly revert to alertness.

Creative Visualization

Creative visualization has been shown to be intensely relaxing. It involves relaxing while envisioning positive, pleasurable mental images. By involving your senses—imagining tastes, smells, textures, and sounds—you build up a rich picture in your mind.

About two billion brain cells make up our speech and thought centers. But our unconscious is made up of 100 billion brain cells, and our visual sense operates mainly in this larger area. No one has figured out why, but our brains don't differentiate between vividly imagined events and real ones. When you think about a painful or frightening situation, your body reacts as though it were really happening, as in the think test (see page 39).

Recent experiments on the muscles of people with back pain showed that muscle tension increased between two and six times when the person being tested simply *thought* about her pain. Reversing this response makes sense. Relaxation with visualization makes a very potent natural relaxant.

To do creative visualization, position yourself as for other methods: sitting comfortably, or lying on your front or back. Bring to mind a pleasurable scene, such as a good memory or one you invent. Remember, for example, a childhood picnic, reliving in detail the sounds of the sea, sun on your skin, sand between your toes, the smell and textures of peeling an orange and its sweet taste.

Other Ways of Relaxing

◆ Yoga classes are an excellent way of combining exercise, breathing, and relaxation. Most classes finish with a 20-minute total body relaxation. Joining a class is a good way for busy people to schedule a time-out without guilt. Shop around to find a class that suits you.

  Avoid the more advanced breathing exercises at first. Stick to low-volume abdominal breathing and explain why to your teacher if asked.

◆ Treating yourself to regular back or full-body massages from a reputable massage therapist is an excellent alternative to the more cerebral approaches to relaxation. Long-term hyperventilators often have stiff, tense upper spines with painful, knotty muscles. Having these gently kneaded back into shape can make you feel you've had three relaxation sessions and a good night's sleep all rolled into one.

◆ Routinely practicing gentle stretches of tense muscle groups is strongly recommended, especially if you have a sedentary job.

◆ Both men and women report the value of having a facial, which includes neck and upper-chest massage. It is also another good way of scheduling a time-out.

♦ Dubbed by one wit as a "wooden Valium," resting in a rocking chair is an excellent quick-fix relaxation method.

How Often? How Long?

Feeling good enough about yourself to take the time to relax is vitally important, and regular practice is a priority in recovery from HVS. The ideal is to weave two 10-minute sessions into your day. Experiment with different methods for different times of the day and week.

You may not feel much immediate benefit, and often it's other people who first remark on changes. It is essential to stick with it. Sometimes at the beginning, unpleasant reactions to "letting go" turn hyperventilators off from continuing with regular practice, but since it is worth persevering, you should try another method.

Regular practice increases your general awareness of stresses and strains and of the need to relax your shoulder and upper-chest muscles. Once you develop an effective relaxation response, "mini-relaxes" practiced several times throughout the day are often sufficient—checking and releasing tension zones as you chest-check your breathing patterns. During the course of the day, check your shoulders, elbows, and hands when walking, making sure they're loose and relaxed.

Just as you recognize triggers that bring on overbreathing, create some relaxation triggers of your own to combat it. Try mentally repeating, "Lips together, jaw relaxed, breathing low and slow," as you turn your palms up and drop your shoulders. Remind yourself how much energy you're wasting by being physically tense, and how continued tension undermines your sense of well-being.

Remember—*relaxation helps eliminate only the symptoms, not the causes of stress.* It's important to develop "the serenity to accept the things you cannot change, the courage to change the things you can, and the wisdom to know the difference"—to paraphrase the Alcoholics Anonymous dictum.

Addiction to bad breathing can be a hard habit to break.

I must admit I thought "relaxation" was a bit too nerdy and navelgazing for me. But when I learned more about the relaxation response and how to switch it on at will without having to lie round going "om" for hours, I was hooked. Short "mini-relaxes" suit my busy lifestyle (which I enjoy) and prevent me from lapsing back into my speedy, hyper ways.

— Barbara, 30

CHAPTER 9

The BETTER Breathing Plan:
T—Talk

Whenever he thought he was about to speak in the tutorial, his breathing lost its regular pattern and he knew it was all over until he could regain control, which would allow his words to come out evenly and without the rushed delivery which made him sound as if he were speaking after a short uphill sprint. . . .

— *From* The Miserables, *by Damien Wilkins*

Coordinating talking and breathing is often a major problem for overbreathers. There are two main reasons for this. The first is that breath control is more difficult while speaking, and the second is that talking about the symptoms and the anxieties associated with HVS often triggers overbreathing.

Breath Control While Speaking

It's important to express ideas and emotions through the power of speech. But the use of quick, gasping upper-chest breaths while talking prompts HVS symptoms.

Slightly husky, light speech, punctuated by throat clearing, sniffing, or yawning, often indicates hyperventilation. Marilyn Monroe's sexy, breathless voice may have had more to do with an overactive upper chest, her waist constricted by a cinch belt restricting normal low-chest breathing. A full-toned, confident voice needs good breath control; ask a courtroom lawyer, actor, or singer.

Try the following techniques to improve breath control while speaking. If you continue to have a problem, get expert advice from a speech therapist. These tips also apply to people who have problems maintaining good breathing while eating.

♦ Relax both shoulders and use abdominal nose-breathing before speaking.

♦ Draw air in through your nose between sentences while talking, instead of quickly upper-chest gasping through your mouth.

♦ Put mental commas and pauses into your speech.

♦ Practice speaking in front of a mirror. Recite the alphabet slowly. Chest-check to observe and correct chest movements.

♦ Practice reading aloud from a book, and tape-record yourself. It's interesting to monitor progress by repeating this every couple of weeks.

♦ Watch other people's breathing patterns when they speak, and listen during telephone conversations. See if you can identify another bad breather.

♦ Be aware of centering your breathing—keep it low and slow.

♦ Combining eating and talking with breathing is a challenge for some. Most of the best advice about relaxed eating was given to us by our parents. Sit down to eat—and avoid eating on the run or talking with your mouth full. This is a fast track to air-gulping and indigestion. Eat very small mouthfuls if "tight throat" symptoms and fear of choking are a problem. Drink small sips to prevent air-gulping. Drinking through a straw is a good way to practice sipping and swallowing.

♦ Never eat while slumped in a low chair; avoid pressure
from the stomach that restricts diaphragm movement.

Repression and Depression

Talking may be particularly difficult when you are voicing
deep anxieties about HVS symptoms.

Bottling up problems is not good for your health. Anxiety
increases mental and physical tension and accelerates adrenaline output. This revs up heart and breathing rates—and HVS
symptoms. Recent scientific research has proved that thinking
or talking about physical symptoms can both directly and indi-
rectly affect your body chemistry.

The indirect physiological effect lies in the relationship
between stress and the onset of exhaustion and depression.
Losing control over parts of your life (as experienced with
chronic hyperventilation) is a major ingredient in some sorts
of depression. A sense of isolation develops if you are afraid of
confiding in anyone. It is worse still if you think of yourself as
neurotic.

Lacking the confidence to handle social events or to keep
up friendships—or thinking you are letting family, friends, or
coworkers down—is a common sign of anxiety and a potent
depressant.

Can You Hear Me?

Listening skills often need brushing up as much as talking
skills; expression and communication are very much two-way
processes. People close to you may have become alarmed,
confused, or even bored by your symptoms.

Relaxing enough to listen closely to other people is as necessary as finding someone who will listen to you.

Deciding to Change

Scientific medicine, with high-tech surgical and pharmaceutical interventions, has revolutionized the healing arts over the last 30 years. But it has also produced an unrealistic belief in a "magic bullet" as the cure-all, encouraging a passive attitude to becoming well. Recovery from hyperventilation requires active involvement and personal commitment. And talking—being able to identify triggers and confront the need for acceptance or change—is a vital part of reducing the stress.

For those who have difficulty identifying the sources of their anxieties, sessions with a clinical psychologist, psychiatrist, or psychotherapist can be of enormous benefit in speeding up recovery.

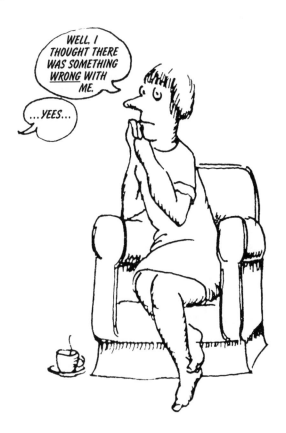

A resonant, confident voice comes with low, slow breathing, relaxation, and talking out—releasing negative emotions. Find someone you trust to confide in. Use positive language. Starting with the next breath, talk yourself up and away from HVS symptoms.

Reading stories to my children is a pleasure now. It used to be a nightmare. I used to read in a monotone without a break, then I'd gasp in a lungful of air and try to carry on. I'd start to feel light-headed. The poor kids—it can't have been much fun for them. We all enjoy it now that I'm breathing properly.

— Elsa, 29

CHAPTER 10

The BETTER Breathing Plan: E—Exercise

When I got back into regular enjoyable exercise, I experienced a conceptual shift in that things that had stressed me out before no longer bothered me. I realized, too, that my inactivity had in itself been a stress.

— Max, 48

Breathing-pattern disorders and low physical fitness levels tend to go hand in hand. This may be due to:

♦ fear of triggering uncontrollable rapid breathing during effort

♦ panic about not being able to breathe in enough air

♦ side effects of poor sleep and exhaustion

♦ fear of fatigue

Nearly all chronic hyperventilators complain of muscle fatigue. The most common types they mention are central fatigue, with general feelings of low energy, and peripheral fatigue felt in the limbs, where muscles tire quickly and ache from lactic acid buildup resulting from low carbon dioxide levels.

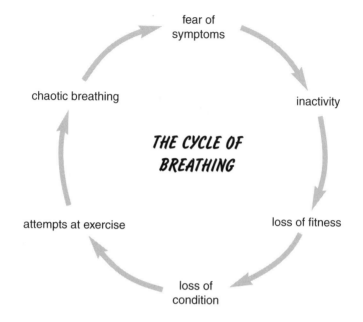

Why Is Physical Fitness Important in HVS?

The effects of inactivity—sluggish circulation, achy muscles, lack of energy, and shortness of breath—not only make you feel below par but add to a general loss of self-confidence.

Fitness is defined as "the body's ability to meet the normal demands of everyday life—work and recreation—with ease, and with enough margin to adequately cope with emergencies." Most hyperventilators would admit falling far short of this description.

Everybody feels better when they have energy to spare. Being fit has added bonuses: it leads to improvement of body image and a stronger sense of self-reliance. Enjoyment of regular physical exercise and the sense of confidence it brings is a vital part of recovery from HVS.

Recent fitness recommendations have changed emphasis from a model of exercise training and fitness to one of physical activity and health "which uniquely incorporates *moderate* intensity and *intermittent* physical activity." This is good news for those who have become drastically inactive or who work long hours in sedentary jobs. It means you can divide up daily physical exercise into short episodes. For example, take a brisk, short walk in the morning, before lunch, and after work.

As long as the accumulated time *gradually* increases towards a total of 30 minutes of brisk activity per day, 6 to 7 days a week, it will provide basic health benefits. For most, this is extremely easy to manage.

Getting Started

Check with your doctor before starting a new activity program.

Start building basic fitness with low-impact exercise options. These include brisk walking, cycling or stationary cycling, low-resistance circuit training, and swimming. Gardening, raking the leaves, mowing the lawn, playing outdoor games with your kids, going dancing, and walking the dog are all excellent "body boosters."

A graduated walking program is a safe, enjoyable, and easy way to improve basic fitness. It's cheap and interesting (looking at your surroundings), and it needs no special clothing except for comfortable walking shoes. A big advantage is being able to nose-breathe while exercising. Invite a friend or partner who knows about your symptoms to "get fit" with you.

(If you don't like outdoor exercise, rent or buy a stationary cycle or a treadmill, and increase your cycling times as you would with walking.)

◆ Set yourself a time, not a distance, to walk (or cycle). Decide for yourself, based on your symptoms, and err on the light side at first. You can start exercising for as little as 3 minutes at a time.

♦ Increase your time by a minute a day or as symptoms allow. Try to do two or three sessions a day until your total exercising time reaches 30 minutes. Hyperventilators tend to be overachievers: make sure your progress is gradual. You can then choose whether to exercise once a day for 30 minutes, or in two 15-minute sessions or three 10-minute sessions per day.

♦ At first, limit yourself to walking on level ground. Make sure your shoulders and arms are loose and relaxed. Use a good arm swing and walk at a brisk pace. As you start to feel fitter and more confident, include slopes and hills. It's normal to puff going up hills—you need more oxygen. Take smaller strides and slow down. Stop and rest if you feel uncomfortable.

♦ If you start to feel breathless or experience chest symptoms, "stop, drop, flop" immediately. Take up a rest position (see page 52). Chest-check and low, slow nose-breathe back to normal before continuing.

♦ Be prepared for ups and downs—some days will be harder than others. Gradually, though, your exercise tolerance and confidence will improve.

When you reach a level where you can manage 30 minutes of brisk exercise a day with little or no symptoms or breathing problems, you have reached a *basic* level of fitness. This will be maintained if you exercise at the same level 6 or 7 days a week.

The joys of walking include:

♦ aerobic benefits (heart/lung efficiency)

♦ improved digestion and bowel function

♦ improved sleeping patterns

♦ relaxation

For variety, include other ways of exercising, such as:

♦ Use the stairs at work. Walk up one flight, or down two, before taking the elevator.

♦ Try a mini trampoline and bounce to your favorite music.

♦ Yoga and t'ai chi classes are especially recommended, combining breathing, exercise (especially flexibility), and relaxation.

♦ Racquet games—tennis, badminton, racquetball, and squash—are great for people needing to release anger, resentment, or frustration.

♦ Join a dance class.

♦ Go swimming or try water jogging. You may need extra help with breathing coordination—check with the instructor.

Eating and Exercise

Good nutrition is an important aspect of fitness, and many authorities cite bad diet as a major source of stress. Not eating properly and not getting enough exercise often go together and lead to physical neglect. This drastically increases the potential for sickness and misery.

If you are overweight, regular exercise helps you lose weight. You feel less like eating directly after exercise, so if you are trying to lose weight, exercising shortly before meals helps tone down the appetite.

If you are underweight, take care to avoid heavy endurance types of exercise and concentrate on flexibility and low-resistance activities well before meals.

Skipping meals and relying on junk foods to boost flagging energy levels will only add to an already overburdened nervous and metabolic system.

Hyperventilators tend to interpret their fatigue as being due to low blood sugar (hypoglycemia). But sugar is not, and never has been, an essential part of our diet. The sugar "high" experienced after eating sweets is short-lived. The body's production of the hormone insulin soon clears the high blood-sugar level and works to restore a normal balance, resulting in a slump in energy. Reaching for more high-sugar food only continues the cycle. Choose protein snacks instead (nuts or cheese), as these keep blood-sugar levels steadier longer. For this reason, a high-protein diet is recommended if you are prone to panic attacks. Experiment and see for yourself.

Alcohol, another high-sugar source, tends to also accelerate the heart rate, fueling overbreathing. While one beer or a glass of wine is an excellent relaxant, more may be asking for trouble.

Smoking

Smoking is another habit that complicates an overbreather's life. It's not hard to imagine the chaos that strong inhalations of smoke wreak upon your already hyperbreathing and overworked upper-chest muscles.

Try to give up smoking while you are retraining your breathing. Join a smoking cessation group. See if you can spot fellow overbreathers.

It's usually more difficult giving up the rituals of smoking, and for hyperventilators that includes that first tidal inhalation after lighting up. Every time you think of the pleasures of smoking, give equal time to acknowledging the harmful effects and what it's doing to your heart and breathing rates. Consider whether you use smoking as an opportunity to hyperventilate. Marijuana smokers are especially prone to doing this.

Think about what sort of smoker you are.

♦ If you smoke to relax, try a "mini-relax" instead.

♦ If you smoke to give yourself a lift, go for a stroll in the fresh air or do some stretches instead.

♦ If you smoke because of the ritual of handling cigarettes and other smoking devices, invest in some worry beads to occupy your hands.

Remember: smoking heavily is asking for trouble. Stopping is best, cutting down helps.

Active Again

Regular enjoyable exercise helps release naturally occurring opioid peptides (endorphins fall under this umbrella) into the bloodstream, and these make you feel good. Bones are kept strong too, which is especially important for those on steroids and for postmenopausal women.

Movement, and pleasure in physical action, are basic human needs. Regular enjoyable activity is very much a part of recovery from HVS.

The combination of loss of fitness and fear of symptoms made me dread the thought of exercise. I used to love running, but after a couple of frightening experiences of shortness of breath, I thought I must have something wrong with my heart. But my heart was fine. My breathing wasn't, though. The cardiologist I saw pointed out my disordered breathing and referred me for physical therapy. I've gradually restored fitness, and I enjoy running again.

— Ted, 47

CHAPTER 11

The BETTER Breathing Plan: R—Rest and Sleep

Sleep: *noun,* the natural periodic suspension of consciousness during which the powers of the body are restored.

— *From* Merriam-Websters Collegiate Dictionary

Rest and refreshing sleep are essential to good health: sound sleep provides a total release from the pressures of daily life. Very few people get through life, however, without from time to time experiencing muddled sleep patterns from extremes of either happiness or sadness. Someone newly in love seems hardly to need sleep at all, and feels no worse for it. But most people find that during periods of stress or sickness the body demands more sleep.

Erratic sleep and vivid or bad dreams are very common hyperventilation syndrome symptoms, and being deprived of satisfying sleep causes a great deal of distress to an already overburdened nervous system. Worrying about symptoms of HVS may be one reason for sleeplessness. But when dreams and nightmares wake you with a pounding heart and in a panic, sleep itself may become feared.

Normal Sleep

Sleep is controlled from a regulating center deep in the brain stem. It processes information from all parts of the body— joints, muscles, organs—as well as from the higher thought

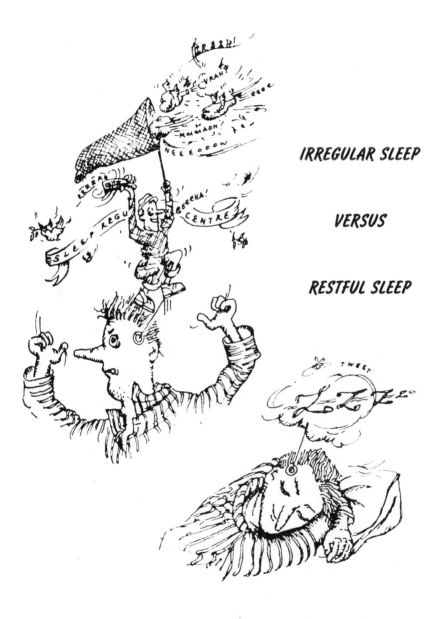

IRREGULAR SLEEP

VERSUS

RESTFUL SLEEP

centers of the brain, or cerebral cortex. A low level of stimulation induces sleep, while a high level of stimulation leads to wakefulness. A calm mind and body are necessary for satisfying sleep.

Sleep goes in cycles. The first main cycle is quiet sleep, which is true rest, with a *quiet* brain. It lasts about an hour. This is followed by rapid eye movement (REM) sleep, a shorter cycle of roughly 20–30 minutes. This is dreamtime, and the brain is *active*.

During quiet sleep the body's metabolic rate, blood pressure, and heart rate lower slightly, and breathing is deep and regular. In REM sleep the heart beats up to 5 percent faster, there is a slight increase in blood pressure and metabolic rate, the eyes dart about under closed lids, and breathing becomes irregular.

The average sleep needed for an adult is $7\frac{1}{2}$ hours— five complete cycles. Individual patterns vary widely according to age, health, and personality.

Why Do People with HVS Have Sleep Problems?

People with HVS are more sensitive to small fluctuations in carbon dioxide levels in their blood. The irregular breathing during REM sleep acts on the unconscious mind, producing vivid or nightmarish dreams and lack of satisfying sleep. Another factor is the respiratory center in the brain, which has become accustomed by day to lower carbon dioxide levels. By night it sends "speed up" signals to the habitual hyperventilator—who may be sinking into relaxed deep breathing during quiet sleep. Feeling sensations similar to the air hunger felt at the start of breathing retraining, the sleeper awakes gasping for air.

Stress levels, high enough during waking hours, are raised further by disturbed rest and the exhaustion caused by poor sleep. Once natural breathing patterns are restored during the day, natural sleep patterns return at night. For some this happens quickly, but for others it takes time and a great deal of patience and understanding to escape the downward spiral of wakefulness, worry, nightmares, and sleeplessness.

Drugs and Sleep

Short courses of antidepressants can be very helpful in restoring a normal sleeping pattern. They help replace chemicals and hormones depleted by stress and lack of refreshing sleep. Some of these drugs are mild muscle relaxants, too, which help reduce physical tension and chronic aches and pains. As they are not physically addictive, be open-minded if this option is suggested.

Sleeping pills are often a blessing for short-lived periods of stress, but if used for more than 2 weeks continuously, they cease to work effectively and become addictive.

If you are dependent on sleeping pills, the information in this chapter will be of little use at first; withdrawal from sleeping pills must be gradual and done with your doctor's help. Use the Good Sleep Plan once you have decided to make a success of getting off sleeping pills.

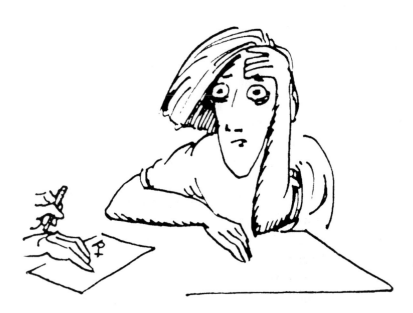

The Good Sleep Plan

Try these simple strategies, and give yourself time to reestablish a refreshing sleep pattern. Let your family and friends know your plans. If you share a bed, your partner will need to know.

Going to Bed

♦ For the duration of sleep retraining (see below), establish regular times to go to bed and get up in the morning. Never go to bed earlier or get up later than these appointed times.

♦ Make your bedroom a stress-free zone. No TV, telephone, noisy clock, personal computer, or radio.

♦ Small changes, such as new bed linens or moving the bed, can help start a new routine and break old associations.

♦ Soft, low lighting creates a restful atmosphere.

♦ Use the bed only for sleeping: no reading, sewing, eating, writing letters, talking on the phone.

♦ Making love is the only exception. Satisfying sex is a powerful prelude to relaxed sleep. Unfortunately, deep postorgasmic relaxation lasts only 4 or 5 minutes, so if you haven't fallen asleep by then, it is of no added benefit. Seek expert help if anxiety about sex is a problem.

♦ Avoid rich, heavy, or late-night dinners or foods high in monosodium glutamate (such as Chinese food) at the end of the day.

♦ Cut out coffee and strong tea for a month (try decaf). Gradually reintroduce it, and even then avoid it after

4:00 P.M. If you're a heavy coffee drinker, be ready for withdrawal symptoms—headaches, irritability, and shakiness. Drink plenty of water.

♦ Avoid TV news and talk radio for a month as well; watch light or funny programs or movies instead. Reduce extremes of positive (late night movies) as well as negative (arguments) stimulation 3 or 4 hours before bed.

♦ Exercise helps reduce stress and induce sleep; if possible, exercise within 4 or 5 hours of bedtime.

♦ Have a warm, not hot, bath or shower before bed. Oil of lavender is an age-old remedy for relaxing mind and body. Add drops to the bath water or on the corner of your pillow.

♦ Cut out daytime naps. Daytime "tiredness" is often the result of boredom or lack of activity. Go for a stroll instead of snoozing.

♦ Try warm milk as a nightcap. Milk has high levels of tryptophan, a naturally occurring enzyme that the body digests and converts into serotonin. This "sleep nectar" has a powerful influence on promoting good moods and sound sleep.

(**Caution:** Tryptophan is an amino acid that was widely used to treat stress symptoms and insomnia. The FDA removed tryptophan from over-the-counter sale in the early 1990s when Japanese manufacturers used a genetically engineered bacterial process to produce tryptophan, leading to eosinophilia-myalgia syndrome. (Belongia 1990)

A plant source of 5-hydroxy-l-tryptophan (5-HTP), the immediate precursor to serotonin (5-hyproxitryptamine), is found abundantly in an African bean (*Griffonia simplicifolia*). Research has confirmed that this form of tryptophan safely converts into serotonin when it reaches the brain and is at least as effective as L-tryptophan in encouraging sleep and reducing anxiety levels. (Zmilacher 1988) 5-HTP is available from health food stores and pharmacists. Read the information leaflets carefully to check for contraindications and possible side effects.)

♦ Sedative herbal teas such as passionflower and chamomile are safe alternatives for those who don't like milk.

♦ Write a list of things to be remembered or done the following day so you don't worry about tomorrow today. Constantly projecting into the future (or past) is a surefire sleep killer.

♦ Avoid going to bed angry.

Getting to Sleep

Based on the sleep-retraining method devised by U.S. physician Richard Bootzin, the following regime has proved extremely successful. Those who have tried this scheme and stuck to it find it takes between 2 and 6 weeks to start working; they also say it is well worth the effort in restoring refreshing, drug-free sleep. You can also try this approach if you wake up during the night.

♦ Once in bed and ready to sleep, lie on your back and practice low, slow abdominal breathing (through the nose) and relaxation techniques. Check tension areas, stretch, and release.

♦ Lie in a comfortable position (usually on the left side to start) and glance at the time.

♦ If after 15 minutes you are still awake, get out of bed. Go into another room and do something else (read, watch a funny video, play solitaire, listen to soothing music).

◆ When you feel ready for sleep, go back to bed, and if
again you are not asleep within 15 minutes, repeat the
sequence until you go to sleep.

**Learn to associate bed with sleep. If you're not sleeping, don't
stay in bed.**

Waking

◆ If your appointed waking time happens to come in the
middle of a deep, quiet sleep cycle, you may find it
hard to wake. Don't interpret this as "waking up
tired." Many admit they let this feeling color their
whole day, but all it means is you've woken from a
deep sleep cycle.

◆ If your appointed waking time comes towards the end
of an REM sleep cycle, you'll wake up more alert,
with fleeting memories of dreams.

◆ If nightmares wake you with hyperventilation symptoms, sit up and recover in a rest position (see page
52). Concentrate on relaxing your neck and shoulders
and on low, slow nose-breathing. When your breathing
and heart rates have slowed, lie down to sleep again,
knowing that overbreathing is the problem and that
you have techniques to combat it.

People who go to bed expecting not to sleep are often
proved right. Breathing control and relaxation reduce tension
and hyperventilation-induced symptoms. Your poor sleep pattern *can* be changed—and a refreshing one restored.

If you continue to have problems, consult a sleep specialist.

It was really strange going for a 6-month checkup after my treatment for hyperventilation syndrome. After going over the list of symptoms I'd had at my first session, I couldn't believe how differently I felt back then. But there it was, all written down. I'm so well now. My sleep patterns are normal; I no longer have those awful symptoms or fears about my health—I've forgotten all about them. It seems when you're unwell that's all you think about. I certainly appreciate feeling healthy again—but, strangely, I don't think about it.

— Trish, 36

WORKBOOK

Commit to Regular Practice

Completing these charts is a graphic way of finding how your stress levels, sleep, and symptom patterns interrelate with each other and with you.

Start with the chart labeled "Identification of Symptoms." This gives you a picture of how you are on day 1, at the start of breathing retraining. On day 1 of week 2, check symptoms again. Repeat on day 1 of week 3.

You can then compare progress from one week to the next. Try not to look at the chart in between times—paper clip the page to the previous one.

Fill in the other charts daily for the next 2 weeks. See if you can identify any patterns.

You should get an idea of what triggers to look out for. Adapt your practice routines accordingly to abolish symptoms.

Identification of Symptoms

Listed here are some typical HVS symptoms. You may have only a few of these symptoms, while others have them all, or vice versa.

Start this chart the day you start breathing retraining. Compare day 1/week 1 with day 1/week 2 and then day 1/week 3.

Symptoms	Example	Week 1	Week 2	Week 3
Chest pains				
Physical tension	√√√			
Tiredness	√√			
Visual disturbances				
Dizziness	√			
Upset stomach	√			
Poor concentration	√√			
Faster or deeper breathing	√√√			
Tight chest	√√			
Feeling revved up				
Tingling fingers				
Sighing/yawning	√√			
Tight jaw/throat	√√			
Headache				
Clammy/cold hands and feet	√			
Erratic/faster heart beats	√			
Others				

√√√ = symptoms all day   √√ = some of the day   √ = intermittent

Which Situations Trigger Breathing Discomfort?

In this chart are listed some situations that may trigger HVS.

Complete the chart, starting on the day you begin breathing retraining, in the same way as you do the "Identification of Symptoms" chart. Compare day 1/week 1 with day 1/week 2 and then day 1/week 3.

Triggers	Example	Week 1	Week 2	Week 3
Driving				
Household chores				
Telephoning	√√			
High humidity				
Kissing/making love	√			
Watching TV/movies				
Talking	√√			
Meetings/interviews	√√√			
Lines/crowds				
Exercise	√√			
Others				

√√√ = always   √√ = often   √ = sometimes

Every morning, afternoon, and bedtime, rate your stress levels by putting a bold dot in the appropriate box. At the end of two weeks, join the dots.

Stress and Strain Gauge

		Day 1			Day 2			Day 3			Day 4			Day 5			Day 6			Day 7	
	am	pm	n	am	pm	n	am	pm	n	am	pm	n	am	pm	n	am	pm	n	am	pm	n
10																					
9																					
8																					
7																					
6																					
5																					
4																					
3																					
2																					
1																					

1 = calm   10 = highly stressed   am = morning   pm = afternoon   n = night

Compare this chart with your "Symptoms," "Eating" and "Sleep" results (see page 98). Is there a pattern?

Stress and Strain Gauge

		Day 8			Day 9			Day 10			Day 11			Day 12			Day 13			Day 14		
		am	pm	n	am	pm	n	am	pm	n	am	pm	n	am	pm	n	am	pm	n	am	pm	n
10																						
9																						
8																						
7																						
6																						
5																						
4																						
3																						
2																						
1																						

1 = calm   10 = highy stressed   **am** = morning   **pm** = afternoon   **n** = night

Symptoms

Breathing Discomfort/Sighing/Air Hunger

Day	1	2	3	4	5	6	7	8	9	10	11	12	13	14
Morning														
Afternoon														
Evening														
Night														

√ = Yes, I am experiencing HVS symptoms   ◯ = I have no HVS symptoms

Eating

Day	1	2	3	4	5	6	7	8	9	10	11	12	13	14
Breakfast														
Lunch														
Dinner														

√ = Yes   ⊠ = On the run   ◯ = Skipped   ⊗ = Upset stomach

Sleep

Day	1	2	3	4	5	6	7	8	9	10	11	12	13	14
# of hours														
# of wakes														
Wake refreshed?														

√ = Yes   ◯ = No

Breathing Retraining/"Time Out"/ Relaxing

Before you get out of bed, lie on your back and nose/ abdominal-breathe for a couple of minutes to establish your breathing pattern for the day.

In bed at night, low, slow nose-breathe while lying on your side to get to sleep.

For the next 2 weeks, schedule time in the morning and afternoon or evening for 10 minutes of relaxed abdominal nose-breathing while lying down. Make it a priority.

Day	1	2	3	4	5	6	7	8	9	10	11	12	13	14
Waking														
Morning														
Afternoon														
Night														

√ = Yes ○ = Forgot/no time

CONCLUSION

Breathing-pattern disorders are alive and thriving in the early twenty-first century.

Definition and diagnosis have been contentious issues in recent years and continue to be the subject of lively international debate. However, enough sufferers have responded to physical therapy interventions involving breathing retraining, relaxation, postural adjustments, and exercise prescriptions, and have enjoyed the far-reaching benefits of balanced blood gases, making following the BETTER Breathing Plan a positive option.

Fifty percent of the cure lies in knowing about and understanding the nature of hyperventilation syndrome. The other 50 percent is a commitment to change.

Use the workbook again and again if you feel symptoms return during times of ill health or stress. Reread the patients' stories and remember you are not alone.

Restoring normal low-chest breathing may take a long time. Don't be too hard on yourself if you do go off the track and lapse back to disordered overbreathing.

Take a break. Take it seriously. Take the next breath low and slow.

Resources

References

Index

Resources

American Association for Respiratory Care

11030 Ables Ln.
Dallas TX 75229-4593
Phone: (214) 243-2272
Website: www.aarc.org
(They have a list of affiliated organizations in the respiratory care area)

American Lung Assocation

1740 Broadway
New York NY 10019
Phone: (212) 315-8700
Website: www.lungusa.org

American Psychiatric Association

1400 K St. N.W.
Washington DC 20005
Phone: (888) 357-7924
Fax: (202) 682-6850
Website: www.psych.org

American Psychological Association

750 First St., NE
Washington DC 20002-4242
Phone: (202) 336-5500
Website: www.apa.org

Anxiety Disorders Association of America

11900 Parklawn Dr.,
Suite 100
Rockville MD 20852
Phone: (301) 231-9350
Website: www.adaa.org

Association for Applied Biofeedback and Psychophysiology

10200 W. 44th Ave.,
Suite 304
Wheat Ridge CO 80033-2840
Phone: (303) 422-8436
Fax: (303) 422-8894
Website: www.aapb.org

References

Chapter 1

Lum, L. C. "Hyperventilation: The Tip and the Iceberg." *Journal of Psychosomatic Research*, vol. 19, 1976.

Magarian, G. "Hyperventilation Syndrome: Infrequently Recognised Common Expressions of Anxiety and Stress." *Medicine*, vol. 64, no. 4, 1982.

Nixon, P. G. F. "Hyperventilation and Cardiac Symptoms." *Internal Medicine*, vol. 10, no. 12, 1989.

Perera, J. "The Hazards of Heavy Breathing." *New Scientist*, Dec. 1988.

Chapter 2

Freedman, R., and S. Woodward. "Behavioural Treatment of Menopausal Hot Flushes." *American Journal of Obstetrics and Gynecology*, 167, 1992.

Hough, A. "Physiotherapy for Survivors of Torture." *Physiotherapy*, vol. 78, no. 5, May 1992.

Schwarztstein, R., et al. "Dyspnoea: A Sensory Experience." *Lung*, 168, 1990.

West, J. B. *Respiratory Physiology* (4th ed.). Baltimore: Williams and Wilkins, 1990.

Chapter 3

Chari, P. "Acupuncture Therapy in Allergic Rhinitis." *American Journal of Acupuncture*, vol. 16, no. 2, 1988.

Ley, R. "Blood, Breath, and Fears: A Hyperventilation Theory of Panic Attacks and Agoraphobia." *Clinical Psychology Review*, 8, 1988.

Widdicombe, J. G. "The Physiology of the Nose." *Clinical Chest Medicine*, 7, 1986.

"The Work, Ways, Positions and Patterns of Nasal Breathing (Relevance in Heart and Lung Illness)." *Proceedings of the American Rhinologic Society*, 1972.

Chapter 4

Gardner, W. N. "The Pathophysiology of Hyperventilation Disorders." *Chest*, 109, Feb. 1996.

Howell, J. B. L. "Behavioural Breathlessness." *Thorax*, 45, 1990.

Chapter 5

Lum, L. C. "Psychogenic Breathlessness and Hyperventilation." *Update*, May 1987.

Timmons, B., and R. Ley, eds. *Behavioural and Psychological Approaches to Breathing Disorders*. London: Plenum, 1994.

Chapter 6

Hough, A. *Physiotherapy in Respiratory Care* (3d ed.). Cheltenham, U.K.: Stanley Thornes Publications Ltd., 2001.

Chapter 7

Jeffers, S. *Feel the Fear and Do It Anyway*. London: Century, 1989.

Ratcliffe, G. *Take Control of Your Life*. Sydney, Australia: Simon and Schuster, 1995.

Chapter 8

Benson, H. *The Relaxation Response*. London: Fount, 1987.

Mitchell, L. *Simple Relaxation*. Edinburgh, Scotland: John Murray, 1988.

Chapter 9

Farhi, D. *The Breathing Book*. New York: Simon and Schuster, 1997.

Smith, G. *Sharing the Load*. Auckland: Random House, 1996.

Chapter 10

Altug, Z., and M. Miller. "The Natural Exercise Prescription." *Clinical Management*, vol. 9, no. 3.

Anderson, B. *Stretching*. Bolinas, CA: Shelter Publications, 1997.

Phillips, Wayne T., et al. "Life Style Activity: Current Recommendations." *Patient Management*, November 1996.

Chapter 11

Belongia, E. "An Investigation of the Cause of the Eosinophilia-myalgia Syndrome Associated with Tryptophan Use." *New England Journal of Medicine*, 323(6):357–365.

Johnston, F. *Getting a Good Night's Sleep*. Auckland: Tandem, 1998.

Zimlacher, K. "L-5-Hypdroxytryptophan Alone and in Combination with a Peripheral Decarboxylase Inhibitor in Treatment of Depression." *Neuropsychobiology* 20(1):28–35.

INDEX

A

abuse victims, 14
accessory muscles, 25–26
African bean, 89–90
age, and hyperventilation
    syndrome, 13
aging, trigger, 36
agoraphobia, 42
alcohol, 82
alkalosis, respiratory, 10, 35
allergies, 33, 38
alternative remedies, 32
altitude, 9
American Association of
    Respiratory Care, 103
American Lung Association,
    103
American Psychiatric
    Association, 103
American Psychological
    Association, 103
amphetamines, 9
anemia, 8
antibiotics, 32
antibodies, 57
antidepressants, 41
antihistamines, 32
anti-inflammatory drugs, 32
Anxiety Disorders Associa-
    tion of America, 103

anxiety, 5, 9, 36, 42
aspirin, 9
Association for Applied
    Biofeedback and Psycho-
    physiology, 103
asthma, 8, 12, 54
autohypnosis, 68
autonomic nervous system, 6

B

bag, paper, 11
BETTER Breathing Plan,
    42–43, 46–92
body mechanics, 60
body temperature, 29
breathing patterns, faulty,
    47–48; normal, 23–34,
    50–51
breathing retraining, 46–55
breathlessness, 5
Buddhism, 10

C

caffeine, 9, 88–89
carbon dioxide, levels in
    blood, 6–8
chamomile, 90
change, 36
chest disease, 8

GET FIT WHILE YOU SIT: Easy Workouts from Your Chair
by Charlene Torkelson

Here is a total-body workout that can be done right from your chair, anywhere. It is perfect for office workers, travelers, and those with age-related movement limitations or special conditions. This book offers three programs. The *One-Hour Chair Program* is a full-body, low-impact workout that includes light aerobics and exercises to be done with or without weights. The *5-Day Short Program* features five compact workouts for those short on time. Finally, the *Ten-Minute Miracles* is a group of easy-to-do exercises perfect for anyone on the go.

160 pages ... 212 b/w photos ... Paperback $12.95 ... Hardcover $22.95

CHINESE HERBAL MEDICINE MADE EASY: Natural and Effective Remedies for Common Illnesses
by Thomas Richard Joiner

Chinese herbal medicine is an ancient system for maintaining health and prolonging life. This book demystifies the subject, with clear explanations and easy-to-read alphabetical listings of more than 750 herbal remedies for over 250 common illnesses ranging from acid reflux and AIDS to breast cancer, pain management, sexual dysfunction, and weight loss.

The author uses no confusing Chinese medical terms and gives sources for all remedies, and there are five indexes to make reference easy. Whether you are a newcomer to herbology or a seasoned practitioner, you will find this book a valuable addition to your health library.

448 pages ... Paperback $24.95 ... Hardcover $34.95

HOW WOMEN CAN FINALLY STOP SMOKING
by Robert C. Klesges, Ph.D., and Margaret DeBon

This guide reveals that what works for men does not necessarily work for women when quitting smoking. Women tend to gain more weight, their menstrual cycles and menopause affect the likelihood of success, and their withdrawal symptoms are different.

Part One guides women in choosing the best time to quit and in deciding which method to use. *Part Two* gives directions for managing withdrawal and weight gain, finding peer support, and controlling stress.

192 pages ... 3 illus. ... Paperback $11.95.

ALZHEIMER'S EARLY STAGES: First Steps in Caring and Treatment *by* Daniel Kuhn, MSW

This book is for the family and friends of those recently diagnosed with Alzheimer's. The first part discusses how the disease affects the brain, known risk factors, the latest treatments, and guidelines for prevention. An important chapter presents what it is like to live with Alzheimer's.

Part Two covers changing relationships, developing new lines of communication, taking responsibility for decisions, and encouraging the patient to try to slow the progress of the disease. Kuhn recommends starting long-term planning immediately and addresses ways that caregivers should take care of themselves.

288 pages ... Paperback $14.95 ... Hardcover $24.95

ALTERNATIVE TREATMENTS FOR FIBROMYALGIA AND CHRONIC FATIGUE SYNDROME: Insights from Practitioners and Patients *by* Mari Skelly and Andrea Helm; Foreword by Paul Brown, M.D., Ph.D.

Many people suffering from fibromyalgia and CFS are unable to find effective treatment and relief. This book combines interviews with practitioners of alternative therapies—including acupuncture, massage therapy, chiropractic, psychotherapy, and energetic healing—with personal stories from patients. These offer a firsthand look at symptoms, treatments, struggles and successes, lifestyle adaptations and medicine, diet, and activity regimens that might help others. There are also sections on obtaining health insurance and Social Security disability.

288 pages ... Paperback $15.95 ... Hardcover $25.95

CHRONIC FATIGUE SYNDROME, FIBROMYALGIA, AND OTHER INVISIBLE ILLNESSES: A Comprehensive and Compassionate Guide *by* Katrina Berne, Ph.D.

A new edition of the classic work *Running on Empty,* this greatly revised and expanded book has the latest findings on chronic fatigue syndrome and comprehensive information about fibromyalgia, a related condition. Overlapping diseases such as environmental illness, breast implant inflammatory syndrome, lupus, Sjogren's syndrome, and post-polio syndrome are also discussed. The book includes possible causes, symptoms, diagnostic processes, and options for treatment.

352 pages ... Paperback $15.95 ... Hardcover $25.95

CREATING EXTRAORDINARY JOY: A Guide to Authenticity, Connection, and Self-Transformation *by* Chris Alexander

Creating Extraordinary Joy takes us on a journey of personal discovery in which we become alive to who we are, where we are in life, and what we value highly. It also helps us conenct to the authenticity and true purpose of others in a condition called "synergy," where the joining of spirit and emotion between two people creates something greater than both.

Using inspirational teachings, images from nature, simple but powerful exercises, and real-life examples, Chris Alexander describes the ten steps of life mastery. Each step yields a life lesson that takes us toward the goals of deepening our passion, opening to abundance, and giving and receiving love. This inspirational guide is more than a book; it is a path to our best self.

288 pages ... Paperback $16.95 ... Hardcover $26.95

THE PLEASURE PRESCRIPTION: To Love, to Work, to Play — Life in the Balance *by* Paul Pearsall, Ph.D.

New York Times Bestseller!

This bestselling book is a prescription for stressed-out lives. Dr. Pearsall maintains that contentment, wellness, and long life can be found by devoting time to family, helping others, and slowing down to savor life's pleasures. Pearsall's unique approach draws from Polynesian wisdom and his own 25 years of psychological and medical research. For readers who want to discover a way of life that promotes healthy values and living, *The Pleasure Prescription* provides the answers.

288 pages ... Paperback $13.95 ... Hardcover $23.95

WRITING FROM WITHIN: A Guide to Creativity and Your Life Story Writing *by* Bernard Selling

Writing from Within has attracted an enthusiastic following among those wishing to write oral histories, life narratives, or autobiographies. Bernard Selling shows new and veteran writers how to free up hidden images and thoughts, employ right-brain visualization, and use language as a way to capture feelings, people, and events. The result is at once a self-help writing workbook and an exciting journey of personal discovery and creation.

320 pages ... Paperback $17.95 ... Third Edition

ORDER FORM

10% DISCOUNT on orders of $50 or more —
20% DISCOUNT on orders of $150 or more —
30% DISCOUNT on orders of $500 or more —
On cost of books for fully prepaid orders

NAME

ADDRESS

CITY/STATE   ZIP/POSTCODE

PHONE   COUNTRY (outside of U.S.)

TITLE	QTY	PRICE	TOTAL
Self-Help ... Hyperventilation ... (paper)		@ $12.95	
Self-Help ... Hyperventilation ... (cloth)		@ $22.95	

Prices subject to change without notice

Please list other titles below:

		@ $	
		@ $	
		@ $	
		@ $	
		@ $	
		@ $	
		@ $	

Check here to receive our book catalog ☐   FREE

Shipping Costs

First book: $3.00 by bookpost, $4.50 by UPS, Priority Mail, or to ship outside the U.S.
Each additional book: $1.00
For rush orders and bulk shipments call us at (800) 266-5592

TOTAL	
Less discount @____%	( )
TOTAL COST OF BOOKS	
Calif. residents add sales tax	
Shipping & handling	
TOTAL ENCLOSED	

Please pay in U.S. funds only

☐ Check ☐ Money Order ☐ Visa ☐ MasterCard ☐ Discover

Card # _____ Exp. date _____

Signature _____

Complete and mail to:
Hunter House Inc., Publishers
PO Box 2914, Alameda CA 94501-0914
Website: www.hunterhouse.com
Orders: (800) 266-5592 or **email: ordering@hunterhouse.com**
Phone (510) 865-5282 Fax (510) 865-4295